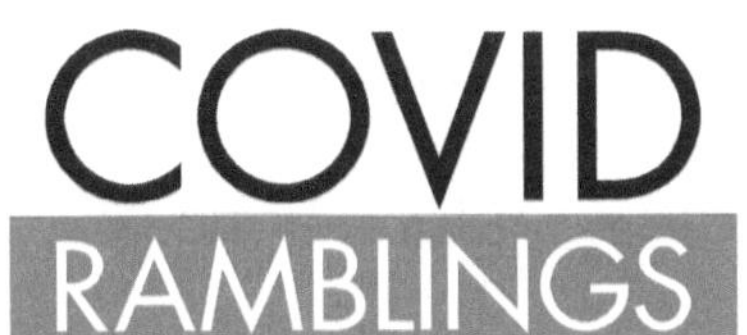
COVID
RAMBLINGS

OTHER BOOKS BY MICHAEL NEVINS

Early Physicians of Northeastern Bergen County

The Jewish Doctor

Jewish Medical Roots

Case Reports: Short Stories About Jewish Doctors

Jewish Medicine. What It Is and Why It Matters

Bergen Pines: A Remembrance of Things Past

Abraham Flexner: A Flawed American Icon

A Tale of Two Villages: Vineland and Skillman, N.J.

Dabrowa: Memorial to a Shtetl

Meanderings in New Jersey's Medical History

More Meanderings in Medical History

Still More Meanderings in Medical History

Meanderings in Medical History: Book Four

Voices From the Bialystok Ghetto

More essays and lectures can be found at michaelnevinsmd.com

COVID

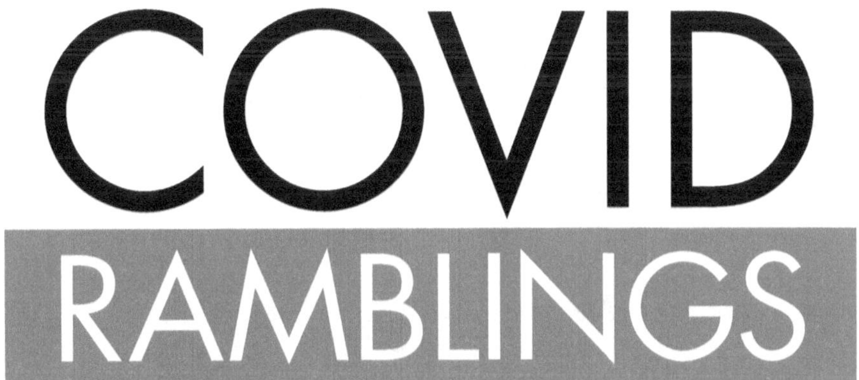

RAMBLINGS

A MEDICAL HISTORIAN DIGRESSES

MICHAEL NEVINS

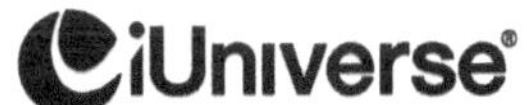

iUniverse

COVID RAMBLINGS
A MEDICAL HISTORIAN DIGRESSES

Scripture taken from the American Standard Version of the Bible.

iUniverse books may be ordered through booksellers or by contacting:

iUniverse
1663 Liberty Drive
Bloomington, IN 47403
www.iuniverse.com
844-349-9409

Because of the dynamic nature of the Internet, any web addresses or links contained in this book may have changed since publication and may no longer be valid. The views expressed in this work are solely those of the author and do not necessarily reflect the views of the publisher, and the publisher hereby disclaims any responsibility for them.

Any people depicted in stock imagery provided by Getty Images are models, and such images are being used for illustrative purposes only.
Certain stock imagery © Getty Images.

ISBN: 978-1-6632-0577-3 (sc)
ISBN: 978-1-6632-0578-0 (e)

Print information available on the last page.

iUniverse rev. date: 08/11/2020

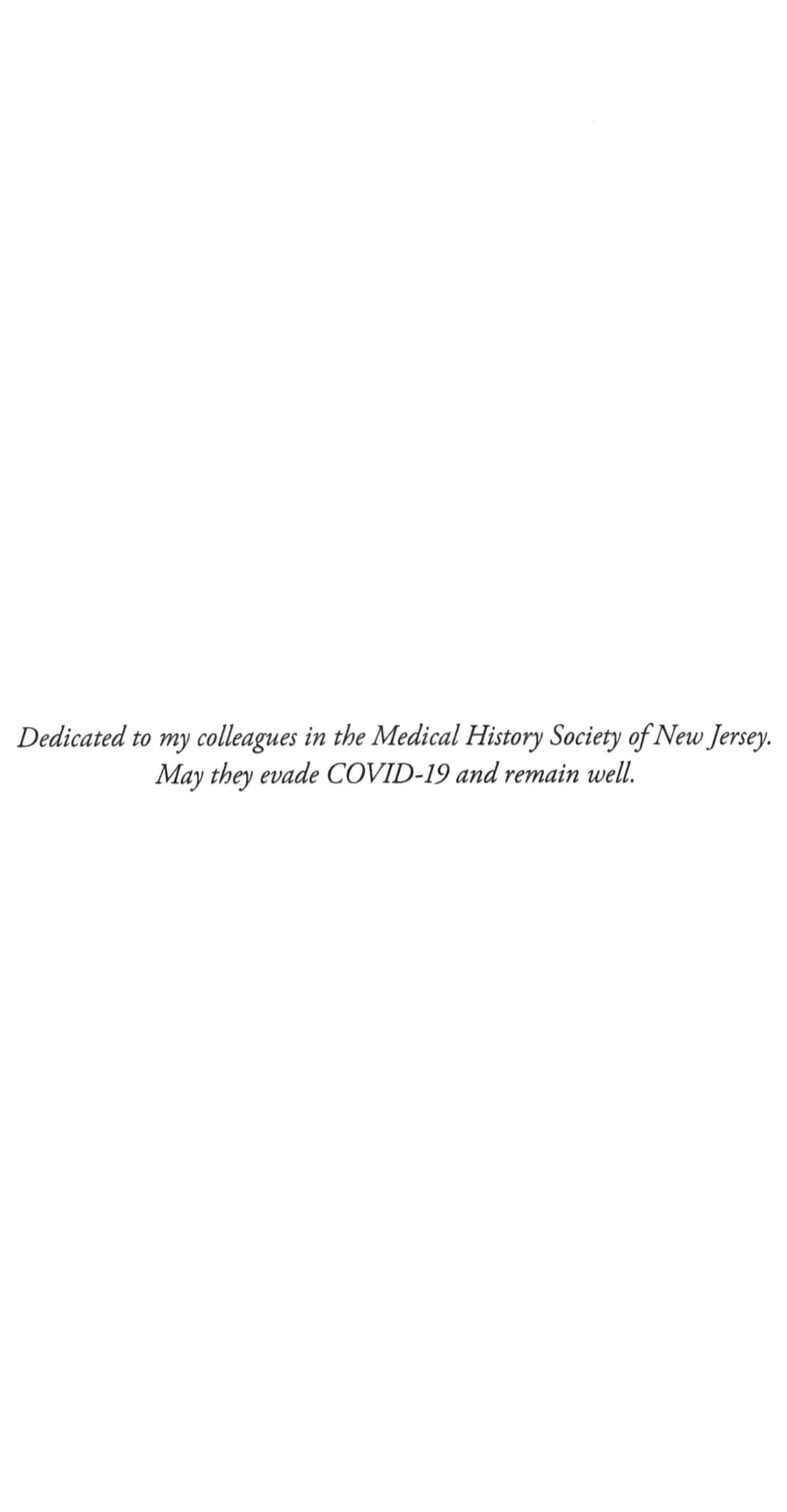

*Dedicated to my colleagues in the Medical History Society of New Jersey.
May they evade COVID-19 and remain well.*

CONTENTS

1

COVID ON MY MIND

I don't know just how or when I was infected but the symptoms began on March 8, 2020: cough, low-grade fever, muscle aches, inability to concentrate and they lasted for about a week. I was sure that I'd caught COVID-19 and, in retrospect, compared to what others experienced it was only a mild case. By the time I finally was able to get my nose swabbed I felt almost normal and then it took another ten days to get the result that confirmed my self-diagnosis.

Although I hadn't altogether dodged the proverbial bullet, it was only a minor flesh wound and after nearly a month of convalescence I felt liberated - free of fear of the dreaded "cytokine storm" that leads to ICUs, endotracheal tubes and worse. Now my army of antibodies was on alert to defend against a return invasion so no worry about reinfection or being contagious to others. Recuperation felt good, but I continued to hand wash frequently and wore my mask in public to show that I was compliant with guidelines - almost as a political statement.

As I slowly emerged from a viral funk, I experienced the same constraints as everyone else: social networking reduced to frequent Zooming, entertainment and dining options virtually non-existent, prolonged idleness and boredom. As an antidote to interminable TV viewing, I resorted to my favorite intellectual hobby: research and writing about medical history. At first I shared some insights with friends and family by e-mail - perhaps to their annoyance - but then a burst of creative energy led to tangential associations that invaded my muddled brain.

Hence each chapter in this brief compendium was prompted by something related to the COVID-19 pandemic which, in turn, led me to recall a subject often far removed from where I began. While digressing, I rejuvenated several oldies from my previous ten books about medical history and added a few newbies. The titles of the last four of my books all included the word *meanderings,* but this time I've chosen to describe these essays as *ramblings.* I really don't know why the change. Perhaps COVID effects the brain. In fact, I'm sure it does and this rather disjointed collection is the evidence.

2
MEMBER OF THE HERD

On everyone's mind during those hectic spring days was how the country, indeed the world, could strike a sensible balance between a healthy economy and a healthy populace. A safe and effective vaccine seemed far off; scientific discovery might be the easiest part and much more formidable likely would be practical matters of production, distribution and cost. Every country was wrestling with the same conundrum and, in the meantime, most opted for cancelling public gatherings and enforcing social isolation.

The outlier was Sweden where everyone was urged to be careful in public and only older adults specifically advised to stay home. Primary schools remained open, people were drinking in outdoor cafes, shopping for clothes, getting their hair cut or styled and enjoying pleasures that Americans were denied. However, Sweden paid a heavy price for this relatively lenient approach. About 30% more Swedes died during the epidemic than is normal at this time of year and more than half were people greater than age 60. As I write, Sweden's per capita death rate is 319 per million compared to 242 per million in the United States. (For comparison, per capita deaths were 91 per million in Denmark, 48 in Finland, 40 in Norway, and 29 in Iceland.) According to the *New York Times*, "Sweden will be judged at the finish line. But it's a very high stakes risk, and the consequences are people's lives."

Swedish authorities hadn't officially declared a goal of reaching "herd immunity," but many scientists believed that would be achieved when more than two thirds of the population has been infected. Some suggested that augmenting immunity might be the only viable defense against the disease and perhaps Sweden was "ahead of the curve." But by late April only 7.3% of people in Stockholm had developed the antibodies needed to fight the disease and when deaths in Sweden rose to five times as many as in their Nordic neighbors combined, Denmark, Norway and Finland closed their borders. Sweden was avoided like the plague.

As the pain of lockdowns grew intolerable, most countries realized that managing, rather than defeating, the pandemic was the only realistic option. It was hoped that as everything started to open up, smart social distancing would keep health-care systems from being overwhelmed and improved therapies for the sickest, and better protections for at-risk groups would help reduce the human toll. However, the elderly and those with immune disorders would remain at great risk. Although for me it felt good to be a survivor, I feared for the rest of my aging herd. Was "the greatest generation" about to be culled?

3

WHAT'S A CORONA?

The dictionary definition of corona is "the rarefied gaseous envelope of the sun that normally is visible only during a total solar eclipse, when it is seen as an irregularly shaped pearly glow surrounding the darkened disk of the moon." By now everyone is familiar with the configuration of the SARS-CoV-2 virus as photographed through an electron microscope, the corona - sometimes called a crown or garland - appearing like a spiky halo that surrounds the molecule.

All well and good but what does this have to do with medical history? I first became aware of the concept way back in the mid-1980s when I was appointed a member of New Jersey's Bioethics Commission. Several years earlier (1976), New Jersey's Supreme Court had ruled in the tragic case of Karen Ann Quinlan that a patient or their representative had the legal right to decline life-preserving medical treatment. That landmark decision altered the balance between doctors and patients from traditional medical paternalism to patient autonomy - the right of an informed patient to decide for him or her self. The Supreme Court's ruling was based on a legal principle of a constitutional right of privacy that had been enunciated eleven years earlier (1965) in still another landmark case, *Griswold v. State of Connecticut.* That case involved a married couple's right to be prescribed contraception and was decided by the United States Supreme Court on the basis of a constitutionally protected right that one's personal information is protected from public scrutiny - what Justice Brandeis once called, "the right to be left alone."

Although the Bill of Rights does not explicitly mention "privacy", Justice William O. Douglas, writing for the majority in *Griswold,* argued that the concept was to be found in the *penumbras* and *emanations* of other constitutional protections, such as the self-incrimination clause of the Fifth Amendment. Penumbra is derived from a Latin word meaning "almost" or nearly" and usually refers to a space of partial illumination as in a solar eclipse. Emanation is defined as an abstract but perceptible thing that issues or originates from a source. There's a difference in meaning, but Justice Douglas seemed to be using the words interchangeably in referring to what he called a *zone of privacy* that's inherent in the Constitution - if not explicit, at least implied - and this concept became a bedrock of American jurisprudence that's often cited in case law.

Coronas, penumbras, emanations - all of these solar references merged in my feverish brain, but why was I worrying about the U.S. Constitution when my personal constitution was being assaulted? Who cares what the virus looks like? I should have been exhorting my B-cells to rev up and destroy the invading bugs. But my mind wandered.

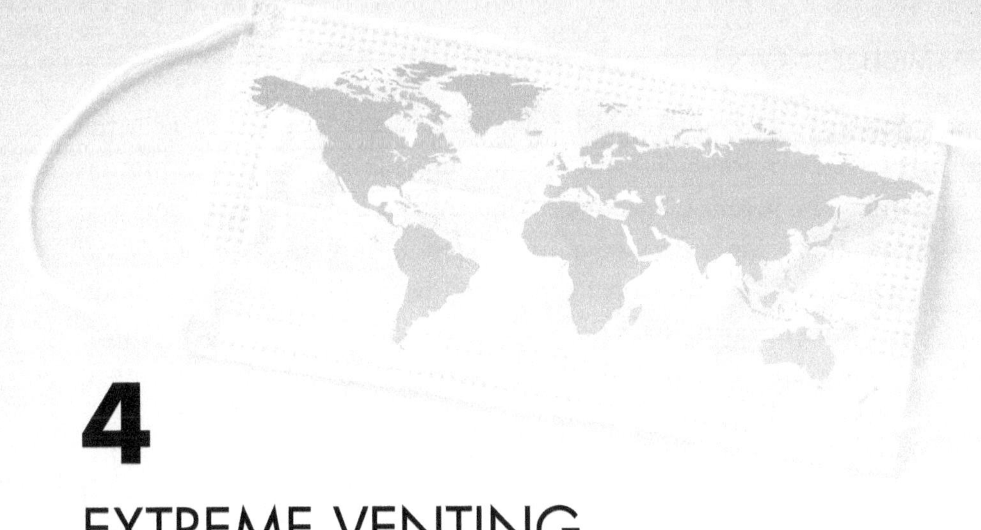

4
EXTREME VENTING
(A long look back)

On several Friday evenings I ventured into Manhattan for dinner with family and experienced a phenomenon that occurred throughout the city every evening at 7:00 p.m. At that precise hour, we leaned out of an open window and joined in a neighborhood cacophony of banging, horn blowing, sirens and shouting. The intent was to express communal thanks for heroic first-responders, but I suspect that it also was therapeutic for everyone, an opportunity to vent frustration after being shut in all day - a primal catharsis. This was distinctly atypical behavior and it reminded me of a very different kind of acting out that occurred in Paris during the 1880s at the giant mental asylum called La Salpetriere. Obviously the two are scarcely comparable but, as explained earlier, the ruminations described herein reflected muddled thinking as I slowly emerged from my encounter with COVID-19.

During the 1880s and 90s, teaching conferences were held every Tuesday morning at La Salpetriere, advertised "to simulate all the surprises, all the complexity of clinical practice." These so-called *Lecons du Mardi* were led by the hospital's medical director, the famous neurologist Jean-Martin Charcot who for many years seemed to bestride the medical world like a colossus. It was as if La Salpetriere was his empire and sometimes Charcot was compared to Napolean or to Julius

Caesar – or to Dante in Hell. He didn't seem to object. In fact, the professor was fond of handing out autographed photos of himself standing Napolean-like with his hand thrust inside his vest. There also was a hint of Greek *hubris* that was evident during the *Lecons du Mardi* when Charcot examined patients suffering from the bizarre condition popularly known as "hysteria."

Since ancient times this wastebasket of symptoms was linked to the uterus – so said the likes of Plato, Hippocrates and Galen. Nervousness, convulsions, contortions, paralysis, anesthesia, frigidity, nymphomania – yes, acting out. Anything that could be lumped together as "female troubles" fit the stereotype. The choking sensation known as *globus hystericus* was blamed on a wandering womb which had migrated up to the throat. Some doctors believed that hysteria was due to sexual deprivation and prescribed vigorous exercise – or more frequent intercourse. But Charcot had mixed feelings about the uterine or ovarian role and gradually came to believe that hysteria was a pathologic brain condition.

Let's imagine that we're entering La Salpetriere's 600 seat amphitheater which was built to accommodate the crowds who clamored to attend – not only physicians, but journalists, theater people, artists, socialites. Every Tuesday morning their carriages clogged the streets of the Left Bank. Something exciting would be happening in this house of horrors: something theatrical or circus-like. There was a hint of scandal for the famous professor was about to open his living museum and display his prize specimens.

At the stroke of 10:00 a.m., Professor Charcot would sweep in, followed by an entourage of interns who referred to him as *le patron*. He was in full command, speaking clearly but not eloquently. The lectures were carefully scripted. Charcot used props to make his points: photographs, plaster models, chalk diagrams on large blackboards. A medical illustrator drew the proceedings and a student transcribed the master's words for publication. But the most important props were the patients themselves. Like marionettes, they were put through their paces by their master puppeteer. They'd been carefully selected by the medical residents to illustrate that day's lesson which during the 1880s most often concerned the clinical aspects of hysteria.

After hypnotizing the women, the solemn professor induced the classic symptoms by pressing on so-called "hysterogenic zones" that had been drawn on their torsos; sometimes he squeezed their bellies using a vice-like instrument called an "ovary compressor." Although he also reported occasional cases of hysteria in men, Charcot insisted that the inciting cause in them was some external trauma such as a fire or accident – in women it was due to something intrinsic, a feminine mystique. For all of his sophistication, Jean-Martin Charcot was a man of his misogynist time when women's emotional behavior seemed inexplicable to men, especially their clamoring for more rights and to be taken seriously. One doctor estimated that one quarter of the women of Paris were hysterics and many doctors had a paternalistic feeling that they had to protect the weaker sex from their own foolish instincts.

Earlier in the 19th century the Continent had been filled with pretenders who claimed to have improved on the experiments of Dr. Franz Mesmer who caused a sensation among high society during the 1780s, just as Charcot would a century later. Mesmer's theory of "animal magnetism" (a universal fluid which effected health and behavior) had been discredited by a royal commission headed by Benjamin Franklin. Employing placebo controlled studies (the first of their kind) it concluded that Mesmer's fashionable "group healings", in which women sat around a large fluid-filled tub, grasped iron wands and listened to soothing music for hours at a time ("mesmerized") were fraudulent.

The 19th century also was a time of well-publicized religious miracles and throughout Europe hypnotism, electrotherapy, hydrotherapy and other fads were being promoted both by sober scientists and charlatans. Mesmer and his followers had given hypnosis a bad name but now the famous Professor Charcot was insisting, not only that it was genuine, but that it was an essential diagnostic tool. To his mind, only true hysterics could be hypnotized, that they had an inherited predisposition that could be unmasked by hypnosis.

To his credit, Charcot wasn't interested in therapeutic miracles so much as putting hysteria on a sound scientific basis. As for therapy, he had nothing special to offer, sometimes sending his private patients to electrotherapists or to Lourdes. As former student Giles de la Tourette would recall, "When I was Charcot's intern, how many times did I hear in the midst of a discussion of my Master's work, 'At La Salpetriere you cultivate hysteria, [but] you don't cure it.'" To which Charcot would respond that before you can cure, you have to learn to recognize.

At the Tuesday morning lessons, Professor Charcot demonstrated what he called the "stigmata" of hysteria: paralysis, contortions, grimacing, shrieking. He had the women bark like dogs, kiss statues or partially disrobe. When he probed their bodies, they responded on cue. They'd learned their parts to perfection for if they did well, they might receive special privileges or presents from the medical residents. The young doctors also wanted to please the professor because their futures depended on his patronage. Journalists suggested that members of the house staff were having love affairs with their patients and probably some were. Those divas who performed best became celebrities and got star treatment. They were painted, sculpted and transformed into characters in operas and novels. Sarah Bernhardt visited to study Blanche's virtuoso performances. It even became chic for society women in *belle époque* Paris to emulate their flamboyant style.

The most famous of all was Blanche Wittman who was called *la reine des hystériques* – the queen of hysterics. As a frightened teenager, she was admitted to La Salpetriere at about the same time that Charcot first became interested in hysteria. She acted out so convincingly that sometimes she was loaned out for display at other teaching hospitals. Her behavior may have reflected addiction to ether which was used on her as a sedative. Two dozen male physicians looked on, seemingly with a mix of interest and desire. After the performance the audience would clap but some critics complained that Charcot was exploiting the women, that the *Lecons du Mardi* were nothing more than a voyeuristic peepshow. But Charcot aimed to demonstrate how susceptibility to suggestion was a cardinal element of hysteria.

This is how one eyewitness described the Tuesday morning scene:

So much has been written and spoken about Salpetriere that there is one name, Charcot, that arouses its own kind of sentiments. Charcot is the sovereign of the kingdom of neuroses. Everyone here relates to him with reverence, bordering on servility. And his appearance actually is as imposing as a general's....The women are treated like cannon-fodder... as if they are medical specimens and nothing more. It never crosses his mind that they might have feelings.

Another insider's description was provided by Jane Avril, the famous cancan dancer at the Moulin Rouge who was immortalized in paintings and posters by Toulouse Lautrec. At age fourteen (1882) she'd escaped from her abusive prostitute mother, was arrested for vagrancy and sent to La Salpetriere. In her memoirs, that were written some fifty years later, Jane Avril recalled the kindness of Charcot's divas who served as surrogate mothers:

I found myself with the stars of hysteria, an ailment which at the time was creating a sensation. The foremost medical men, the best known thinkers of the entire world came in droves to attend the courses presided over by the master and to witness the demonstrations and experiments on his most famous subjects. They were deranged girls whose ailments named Hysteria consisted, above all, in simulation of it. How much trouble they used to go to in order to capture attention and gain stardom....

The prize went to the one who would find something needed to overshadow the others when Charcot, followed by a large group of students, stood at the bedside and observed their wild contortion, various acrobatics and other gymnastics. These patients had nothing to hide from little me I was of so little consequence – thus they didn't

> *hesitate to let me know about what they used to call "the*
> *secret."*

Jane Avril stayed at La Salpetriere for eighteen months and just before discharge she attended the annual masquerade ball which was called *La Bal de Folles* – the Madwomen's Ball. That night Jane was a sensation, kicking up her heels and gesticulating wildly and as soon as she was released, she went straight to Montmartre, got a job dancing at the Moulin Rouge and became the toast of the town and the inspiration of Toulouse Lautrec.'

Charcot was a heavy cigar smoker and a gourmand and died of heart failure in 1893 at age 68. Once he was gone, the so-called "Salpetriere School" fell like a house of cards. Rivals froze his former residents out of academic appointments and the idea of hysteria being a distinct neurologic condition was dismissed. The 1880s sometimes were described as "the Golden Age of Hysteria" and, if so, La Salpetriere was the epicenter. Twenty years before Charcot had arrived in 1862, only 1% of the hospital's inmates carried this diagnosis; during his heyday 17% did and twenty years after his death, there were none.

Back in Vienna, his former pupil Sigmund Freud recalled how at one of the weekly soirees held at Charcot's elegant home, he'd overheard the master explain to someone, "c'est toujours la chose genital, toujours, toujours, toujours" and when he heard this revelation, "I was paralyzed with astonishment." So it was in Paris that Freud first came to appreciate that physical signs and symptoms could have a psychologic basis and that repressed sexual events could be the basis of neuroses. He expanded on this insight for the next fifty years.

Whereas during the 1880s Charcot's hysterical divas acted out every Tuesday morning in Paris, in a very different manner in 2020 so do home-bound Manhattanites every evening at 7:00 p.m. To be sure, the reason for and nature of their exuberant performances differed markedly, but for each of the participants there was a common sense of release and exhilaration. *Vive la différence!*

5

ISOLATION

Everyone was frustrated by the need for physical distancing and staying at home as the best ways to reduce the spread of COVID-19. Although requirements varied between states, they were not nearly as severe as monitored "lock-downs" that were imposed in some other countries. During idle hours alone at home, my mind sometimes drifted to a much earlier time when social isolation and inactivity was thought to be an effective form of medical treatment, in some quarters even considered to be fashionable.

If Jean-Martin Charcot was France's leading neurologist during the late 19th century, his equivalent in the United States was Philadelphia's S.Weir Mitchell (1829-1914). Like Charcot, Dr. Mitchell was a student of diseases of the mind. However, his favorite was not hysteria but an ill-defined condition called neurasthenia that was characterized by such vague symptoms as fatigue, headache, insomnia, indigestion and irritability that seemed to be especially prevalent in women. For them, during the 1870s, Weir Mitchell devised what he called the Rest Cure. (By contrast, nervous men were encouraged to engage in vigorous activity out West.)

The Rest Cure was highly regimented. In it Dr. Mitchell strove for an atmosphere of "order and control" that would serve as "moral medication" for coddled invalids. Wealthy women from near and far flocked to Philadelphia. A patient was not allowed to read, write, sew, feed herself or have contact with friends or family. She had to lie down in bed for six to eight weeks and needed the doctor's permission to sit up in bed or turn over without assistance. Massage and electrical stimulation ensured that muscles didn't atrophy. The diet was gargantuan: huge portions of meat, three or four pints of milk drunk at and after meals, supplements of iron, strychnine, arsenic and cod liver oil. Women who refused might be force fed through the nose or rectum, sometimes whipped to ensure obedience. As Dr. Mitchell wrote, "a gain in fat up to a certain point seems to go hand in hand with a rise in all other essentials of health."

One of Weir Mitchell's patients was the author and social activist Charlotte Perkins Gilman who underwent the Rest Cure in 1887 during a bout of postpartum depression. It seems that she got off relatively easy compared to the regimen just described. She explained in her autobiography:

> *I was put to bed and kept there. I was fed, bathed, rubbed, and responded with the vigorous body of twenty-six. As far as he could see there was nothing wrong with me, so after a month…he sent me home with this prescription: "Live as domestic a life as possible. Have your child with you all the time…Lie down an hour after every meal. Have but two hours intellectual life a day. And never touch pen, brush, or pencil as long as you live."*

After faithfully following this prescription for several months, Charlotte Gilman wrote that she was "perilously near to losing my mind. The mental agony grew so unbearable that I would sit blankly moving my head from side to side." In 1892 she published a semi-autobiographical short story called *The Yellow Wallpaper*, in which she condemned the Rest Cure and by extension the harmful treatment of women by male physicians. From Gilman's perspective Weir Mitchell was a medical misogynist and the Rest Cure was Gothic torture.

The narrator in *The Yellow Wallpaper* described how after the birth of her first child she became increasingly nervous and depressed. Her husband, who also was her doctor, confined Charlotte to a nursery in hopes that "perfect rest" would restore her to health. When her recovery stalled, he threatened a more drastic treatment. As she related, "If I don't pick up faster he will send me to Weir Mitchell…but I don't want to go there at all." Entirely shut off from social contact or diversion, she became obsessed by the room's yellow wallpaper and nearly turned psychotic.

Nowadays when we're in social isolation we have many ways to maintain contact with the outside world, but one thing that resembles Weir Mitchell's Rest Cure is what some people call "quarantine weight." Some people insist that the "19" in COVID-19 should refer to the quantity of adipose gained as a result of turning to food to help cope with anxiety and boredom (instead of to 2019, the year of the first case.) I presume that applies equally to men as to women.

6

MIRACLE DRUG
(For Physicians)

At the urging of the well known medical expert Donald J. Trump, who called it "a game changer," the FDA approved the combined use of the arthritis drug hydroxychloroquine (HCQ) and the antibiotic azithromycin for emergency use to treat COVID-19. Later the agency reversed its self but the president remained adamant and began using HCQ prophylactically. After all, he argued, it couldn't hurt so there was nothing to lose. Perhaps it helped DJT's bone spurs, but it's extremely unlikely that HCQ was effective as an anti-viral agent. When TV pundits and journalists warned about the drug causing ominous cardiac arrhythmias, as a retired cardiologist I decided to explore the available evidence for my self.

In order to understand the matter one has to be knowledgeable about electrocardiography which is a challenge even for physicians. To be sure, each of the drugs in question may be associated with prolongation of the QT interval, which on rare occasions may lead to a potentially fatal form of ventricular tachycardia. The French have a catchy description for it called *torsade de pointes* (TdP) translated as "twisting of peaks." That's because the ECG pattern exhibits a distinctive cyclic shifting of the QRS axis from positive to negative and back.

The QT interval is the time from the beginning of the QRS complex that represents ventricular depolarization to the end of the T wave which represents repolarization. The measurement frequently is corrected for the effects of heart rate to produce what's referred to as QTc. A normal interval is up to 400 milliseconds and greater than 500 is grounds for concern. Yes, I know, these are relatively arcane details but what's important is that a prolonged QT interval is potentially arrhythmogenic and can serve as an imprecise metric for drug safety. Several electrolyte and metabolic abnormalities beside drug effects also can affect the QT interval.

Chloroquine and its derivative hydroxychloroquine have been in clinical use for more than a half-century as an effective therapy for treatment of some malarias, lupus, and rheumatoid arthritis. (In this DJT was correct.) Although data show mild QT prolongation associated with both agents, several hundred million courses of chloroquine have been used worldwide making it one of the most widely used drugs in history, yet without reports of arrhythmic death from the World Health Organization or from rheumatologists who've been prescribing chloroquine or HCQ for many years.

By the middle of May, there was very little published information available on-line from which to extrapolate cardiac risk. A report from Brazil (*Journal of the American Medical Association,* April 24, 2020) described results of a double-blind, randomized clinical trial that tracked 81 adult patients hospitalized presumably with COVID-19. 40 patients were given 450 milligrams of chloroquine twice on the first day and once every day for the following four days while 41 others were given 600 milligrams twice daily for 10 days. All patients also were given azithromycin. By day 13, six patients in the low-dose group had died, as did 16 in the high-dose group. Preexisting heart abnormalities were present in 11 of the 81 patients and two of the 41 patients in the high-dose group experienced ventricular tachycardia.

In that study, because of delays in testing for the virus, chloroquine treatment was initiated based on suspicion of COVID-19 but, ultimately, only 31 of 40 patients (77.5%) in the low-dose group and 31 of 41 patients (75.6%) in the high-dose group tested positive for the virus

Prolongation of QTc interval was observed in 4 of 36 patients (11.1%) in the low-dose group and 7 of 37 patients (18.9%) in the high-dose group and two of these experienced ventricular tachycardia. By day 13 of enrollment, 6 of 40 patients (15.0%) in the low-dose group had died, compared with 16 of 41 patients (39.0%) in the high-dose group, but there was no evidence of death associated with prolonged QTc nor any witnessed instances of *torsade de pointes.*

An editorial in the *Journal of the American Medical Association* that accompanied this Brazilian study concluded that high-dose chloroquine (and by association, hydroxychloroquine) in combination with azithromycin may be associated with increased mortality among patients with severe COVID-19 but not necessarily as a result of a drug-related arrhythmia. Concerning cardiac toxicity from azithromycin alone, the literature has provided conflicting information. In a review of 12 case reports of fatal arrhythmias in patients receiving the drug there was no significant relationship between dose and QTc interval duration and all 12 had at least two additional risk factors.

A retrospective observational study of outcomes of more than 1,400 COVID-19 patients from multiple hospitals in the New York Metropolitan area (*JAMA* on-line, May 11) compared the incidence of abnormal electrocardiograms (arrhythmias or prolonged QT) and cardiac arrests in four groups: patients receiving HCQ + azithromycin (22.1% abnormal ECGs, 15.5% cardiac arrests), HCQ alone (27.3%, 13.7%), Az alone (16.1%, 6.2%), neither drug (14%, 6.8%.) Differences were statistically significant only for the combination. Overall, treatment with hydroxychloroquine, azithromycin, or both was not associated with significantly lower in-hospital mortality nor ECG abnormalities.

A report from China of 150 hospitalized patients from 16 centers found HCQ didn't help clear the virus or relieve symptoms for COVID-19 patients any more than standard care alone and it had more side effects. Adverse events were reported in 8.8% of patients in the control group compared with 30% in the HCQ group but no cardiac arrhythmias were reported. (Diarrhea was the most common side effect, occurring in 10% of patients in the HCQ group vs none in the control group.)

In another study of 84 patients with coronavirus who received HCQ, 30% developed minor QTc prolongation which in 11% exceeded 500 milliseconds. But there were no cases of VT. An earlier report from China in 2006 described an elderly woman with lupus who took HCQ long term and developed refractory ventricular tachycardia (TdP). When the drug was stopped her QT shortened and heart rhythm normalized. Such anecdotes aside, lethal ventricular tachycardia does not appear to be a frequent complication of these drugs. Still another article (*Lancet,* May 22) combined data from 671 hospitals on six continents. 15,000 out of 96,000 patients received either chloroquine or HCQ alone or combined with an antibiotic like azithromycin and hospital mortality was greater in those patients receiving some combination of these drugs, 1 in 6 compared with 1 in 11 in controls. QT intervals weren't reported but there was increased incidence of ventricular arrhythmias (6.1% with HCQ alone, 4.3% with chloroquine alone and 6.5% when one of them combined with the antibiotic.) vs. 0.3% in those not receiving them.

When both the American Heart Association and American College of Cardiology warned against routine use of hydroxychloroquine for treatment of COVID-19, a deluded FOX newscaster proclaimed that taking HCQ is akin to a death sentence! Nevertheless, Dr. Trump remained enthusiastic and seemed to be tolerating it. On June 15 the FDA revoked emergency authorization for these malaria drugs amid growing evidence that they didn't work against the virus and could cause serious side effects. As a result the federal government was stuck with 63 million doses of hydroxychloroquine that it began stockpiling after President Trump touted it as "very encouraging" and "very powerful" and a "game-changer."

In May two prestigious medical journals (The Lancet, May 22, and New England Journal of Medicine, May 1) published articles by the same author suggesting that patients treated with hydroxychloroquine were at high risk of serious cardiac arrhythmias, but later, both papers had to be retracted because of faulty data collection. By late June, there was a second wave of enthusiasm for the anti-malaria drug with President Trump still vigorously promoting it as a possible cure for Covid-19.

7

PERSONAL SPACE

In this Age of COVID, the dimension six feet has taken on crucial significance as the distance that defines relatively safe separation from other peoples' pathogens. Beyond strictly microbiological considerations this finite distance also can be understood metaphorically - and even Jewishly. In 1981 I composed an essay titled "Jewish Space" in which I noted that the Talmud often cited specific rules that involved linear measurement. It seems apt today.

The basic unit in ancient times was the cubit, defined as one forearm's length - roughly 18 inches from elbow to tip of index finger. Indeed, *four cubits equaled six feet* and was a dimension that appeared with some frequency. For example, any unclaimed object found within four cubits of a person is legally his; or if a man throws a divorce writ within four cubits of his wife she is officially divorced; if a man "breaks wind" while saying the *Sh'ma* he is obliged to move away four cubits before continuing.

Four cubits defined personal space that extended beyond one's corporeal self and sometimes had meaning beyond the strictly legal. For example, when Moses commanded (*Exodus* 16:28) that on the Sabbath "Let not any man go forth from his place" this evoked various rabbinic opinions. One was that although on the Sabbath a Jew is prohibited from walking more than 2,000 cubits beyond the town limits, some he could go precisely four cubits more. Why? Because that is equivalent to one's personal space, his or her "turf." It's like a bubble that surrounds the individual, violation of which may induce psychologic or physiologic stress - or during a pandemic might cause contagion.

At times Jewish thought appears to box itself into a corner by virtue of excessive rigidity, but it also is capable of turning a seeming contradiction to its advantage. Consider the mob scene in the Temple on high holy days when all of the Israelites were crowded together. Wouldn't this have created an intolerable mass violation of the doctrine of four cubits of personal space? Not necessarily. In "The Sayings of the Fathers" (*Pirke Avoth*) a collection of ethical words of wisdom of the sages, included among ten miracles that were associated with the Sanctuary is this fact: "Although the people stood closely pressed together, they found ample space to prostrate themselves." It's been suggested as explanation for this conundrum that when people stood straight, unbending and proud, there would be sufficient space; but when they humbled themselves by bowing to G-d, *miraculously* there would be space enough. So the sages were not above using a little magic for a good moral cause. One wonders how they would have dealt with the coronavirus?

The Torah understood the concept of cleanliness and contagion and required that lepers be strictly isolated: "All the days wherein the plague is within him he shall be unclean; he shall dwell alone: without the camp shall his dwelling be." (*Leviticus* 13:45-46). Nevertheless, lepers were permitted to pray in synagogue, but they had to enter and leave separately and were confined to a railed off section ten handbreadths high and *four cubits* wide in order to ensure public health.

Jewish thought characteristically is oriented toward the real world rather than the abstract, so it should not be surprising that law and literature often are expressed in physical terms and contain metaphors referring to space, both personal and cosmic, inner and outer. In the modern era Rabbi Abraham Joshua Heschel declared that time is more important than space and argued that the Sabbaths are "our great cathedrals…the architecture of our time." And in his book *The Sabbath*, the poetic rabbi pleaded against man's unconditional surrender to space, meaning his enslavement to things. Spatial metaphors illustrate the subtlety of Jewish thought but also can serve to illuminate its moral content.

Whether you prefer the familiar tried and true dimension six feet or the ancient four cubits to describe our personal boundaries, it's best for each of us to manage our space both figuratively and metaphorically. Amidst the current pandemic, even as we fixate on practical matters, now is an opportune time for us all to consider implications of the global disaster in a broader context than our physical isolation. Our mutual challenge is to shun stagnation and remain engaged in events beyond our physical enclaves - and to make our voices heard.

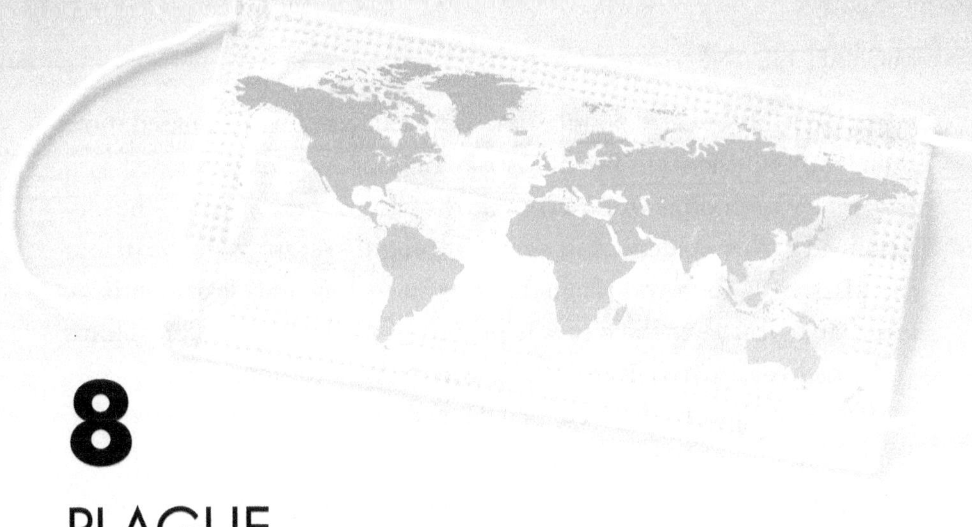

8

PLAGUE
(The more things change the more they are the same)

The ancient Greeks called any human scourge "plague" - from the word *plaga*, meaning a blow. There was a severe outbreak that began in 541 A.D. followed by repeated recurrences over the next two centuries. In Renaissance Europe plague was a constant nightmare and many people believed that it represented Divine punishment. Mention the word and people would make the sign of the cross and say "God deliver us from it." Once plague came it remained endemic for centuries with cyclic flare-ups. The notorious Black Death ran from 1347 through 1352 and decimated between 25 and 75 million Europeans, best estimates being more than one third of the population.

Bocaccio reported that the wealthy of Florence found refuge in palaces "removed on every side from the roads [with] wells of cool water and rare wines." The title "Black Death" didn't come into use until the 15th century and it remains unclear whether the adjective was meant to describe the characteristic blue-black rash and terminal cyanosis or as a general comment on the dismal times. When pandemics flared up they were devastating not only to the population but had enduring effects on the economy, politics and culture.

Compared to the Black Death London's cataclysm in 1665 was relatively minor. The scarcely reliable official figure was 68,596 deaths, nearly 20% of the city's population; some scholars have estimated more than 100,000 victims. Pre-industrial London was overcrowded and unsanitary with offal and excrement thrown into the streets. The city sustained earlier epidemics in cycles of roughly six to twelve years but the disaster of 1665 was plague's last gasp in England. Providentially, less than a year later the city was purged of its disease-breeding slums and largely destroyed by an inferno which raged for four days.

Even the most educated people had no idea of its true cause: something in the air, weather conditions or natural phenomena such as earthquakes, comets or misalignments of the planets. Fires were burned in London's streets to clear the air and in sickrooms to destroy the clothes of victims. Because tobacco was thought to be protective, schoolboys at Eton were forced to smoke and those who disobeyed were flogged. Some blamed the sickness on dogs and cats but their mass slaughter was counterproductive - after all, cats killed rats which carried fleas which, in turn, were the actual transmitters. Others sought human scapegoats. (Infamously, during the Black Plague of the 15th century Jews had been accused of well-poisoning which led to murderous pogroms.)

Madmen roamed London's streets prophesying doom and the city became a vast mortuary; according to one observer "a reeking prison house of the living, the dying and the dead." The only commerce that thrived was grave-digging but the diggers were quickly overtaxed. Church bells tolled night and day. Those who could fled the cities - a mass exodus of some 200,000 out of a half-million Londoners. To discourage refugees, walls were built around cities and their gates locked. Panicked itinerants had to bribe to gain entry while vigilantes armed with pitchforks and muskets guarded the roads. For the benefit of those left behind during the exodus, the College of Physicians, fifty of the medical elite, the great majority of whom evacuated London, issued a manual called *Certain Necessary Directions for the Prevention and Cure of the Plague.* It advised shut-ins to think pleasant thoughts of gold and silver rather than to brood about death.

Both the afflicted and their families were confined to their homes which then were locked and marked by a red cross. Sealed off from the outside world, these charnel houses were closely guarded; keyholes were plugged to keep the "miasmic" air inside so as not to endanger passers by. Medical supplies and food would be passed through a window by a courier. Although the municipality or the church were supposed to provide for the poor, the unaffected were unwilling to be taxed to pay for those locked in the penthouses nor for those assigned to attend them. The famous diarist Samuel Pepys acknowledged that the plague "makes us cruel, as dogs, one to another." Nevertheless, harsh methods were necessary to preserve the greater good in dangerous times: "But Lord! How sad a sight it is to see the streets empty of people."

Physicians, surgeons and apothecaries were equally impotent as the quacks, mountebanks and melange of alternative healers. Most so-called "plague doctors" were not really physicians but municipally employed inspectors whose prime function was to count the dead in the pest houses. They wore floor-length leather or oil cloth robes (the filthy plague atoms were thought to catch on to coarse wool or cotton fibers) which attracted rather than repelled rat fleas. Their faces were protected by fearsome masks with bird-like beaks which were stuffed with a mixture of aromatics, not only to counter the repugnant odors but to combat air-borne poison. Bills of Mortality were circulated every week that charted the number and locations of the dead and buried.

According to ancient Galenic principles, the humors had become unbalanced by corruption which called for strong applications of whatever might eliminate the putrid matter, including bleeding and blistering. In 16th century Provence, the famous prophet-physician Nostradamus disapproved of bleeding, recommending instead nourishing food, clean bed linens and fresh air. That was good advice but Nostradamus also devised his own prophylactic formula urging people to suck a lozenge which he concocted mainly out of rose petals. Although he touted this as a panacea, alas, it was insufficient to save the prophet's own family.

Daniel Defoe was no more than age six in 1665 when the pestilence appeared in London; too young to remember many details but old enough to hear and read firsthand reports of others. He was a prolific writer with more than 370 publications - the most famous being *Robinson Crusoe*. In 1722, when he was in this sixties, Defoe published *A Journal of the Plague Year,* supposedly a newly discovered eye-witness account;

the subtltle noted that it was written by "a citizen who continued all the while in London and never made Publick before."

By the time that Defoe wrote the journal, he was beset by debt, pilloried for his political leanings and had a wife and seven children to support. At the same time there was national panic about events in Marseilles in 1720-21 when there were more than 50,000 deaths during the last great epidemic in Europe. The English feared that the Great Plague might come again and from their pulpits, ministers urged parishioners to repent. Capitalizing on public anxiety Defoe's more than 200 page allegedly eye-witness recounting of London's earlier experience was a guaranteed best seller. What follows next are slightly edited selections which depict the horror much more colorfully than the drab prose of proper historians.

> *The nobility and gentry thronged out of town with their families and servants…Indeed nothing was to be seen but wagons and carts with goods, women, servants, children, &c; coaches filled with people of the better sort and horsemen attending them and all hurrying away… all loaded with baggage and fitted out for traveling…This was a very terrible and melancholy thing to see and it was a sight which I could not but look upon from morning to night, it filled me with very serious thoughts of the misery that was coming upon the city and the unhappy condition of those who would be left in it.*

> *This hurry continued for some weeks, that is to say, all of May and June, and the more because it was rumored than an order of the government was to be issued out, to place turnpikes and barriers on the road to prevent people's traveling; and that the towns on the road would not suffer people from London to pass, for fear of bringing the infection along with them., though neither of these rumors had any foundation but in the imagination, especially at first.*

I had two important things before me: the one was the carrying on my business and shop, which was considerable, and in which was embarked all of my life in so dismal a calamity…I went home greatly depressed in my mind, irresolute and not knowing what to do. I had set the evening wholly apart to consider seriously about it and was all alone; for already people had, as it were by a general consent taken up the custom of not going out after sunset.

From the moment that I resolved that I would stay in town…casting myself entirely upon the goodness and protection of the Almighty, I was in his hands,, and it was meant he should do with me as should seem good to him. With this resolution I went to bed and I was farther confirmed in it the next day by the woman being taken ill with whom I had intended to intrust my house and all my affairs.….It was a very ill time to be sick in for if one complained it was immediately said he had the plague; and though I had indeed no symptoms of this distemper, yet being very ill, both in my head and in my stomach, I was not without apprehension that I really was affected - but in about three days I grew better.….the apprehensions of it being the infection went quite away…and I went about my business as usual.

Daniel Defoe described how wandering beggars were banned from the streets and how "plays, bear-baitings, singing of ballads, disorderly tippling" all were prohibited. Each parish would select a few persons "of good sort and credit" to serve as "examiners" for at least two months. Those who declined were committed to prison until they relented. Their role was to visit each home and report plague victims to the constable who would have the house shut up for at least four weeks "after all be whole."

Watchmen kept the keys and ensured that no one went in or our "upon pain of severe punishment." Necessities might be brought to shut-ins by the watchmen "at their own charges, if they be able, or at the common charge if they are unable." Unfortunately, these watchmen came from the lowest levels of the social order and frequently were drunk, boorish or indifferent to the welfare of those they were supposed to protect. If the family starved to death, the watchman still earned his wages. In addition to the watchmen, every parish appointed women searchers "of honest reputation and of the best sort as can be got in this kind" to ascertain whether the dying or dead truly were plague victims and to advise officials in order to permit an accurate body count. During their employment, searchers were not permitted "to use any public work or employment or keep any shop or stall or be employed as a laundress" lest they spread infection.

A small number of chirurgeons (surgeons) were assigned to check the accuracy of the searchers' findings, each to be paid twelve pence a body searched by them "out of the goods of the party searched, if he is able, or otherwise by the parish." Because it was feared they might spread infection when walking in the streets, searchers, chirurgeons, keepers and buriers had to hold "a red rod or wand, three foot in length, in their hands and evident to be seen." When not at work they were to enter no house but their own and "to forbear and abstain from company, especially, when they have been lately used in any such business or attendance."

One of the few physicians who didn't desert London, Dr. Nathaniel Hodges was hired by the government for a stipend of 100 pounds for "the prevention and cure of the plague within the city" and later published his own account in which he described how he conducted house calls. "I kept in my mouth some lozenges all the while I was examining them. I took care not to go into the rooms of sick when I sweated or was short-breathed with walking, and kept my mind as composed as possible, being sufficiently warned by such who had grievous sugared by uneasiness in that respect."

Dr. Hodges doubted the wisdom of quarantine measures since placing a red cross on the door caused neighbors to flee, depriving the sick of their assistance; keeping people shut up without access to fresh air and exercise also made no sense: "Liberty is necessary for the comforts both of body and mind." Hodges' most scathing criticisms were directed at "the wicked practices of nurses, not to be mentioned but in the most bitter terms…these wretches, out of greediness to plunder the dead, would strangle their patients and charge it to the distemper in their throats. The doctor claimed that one man was stripped of his clothes and money and left to die, only to recover after the nurse left.

Nathaniel Hodges had his own preventative remedy: every morning he took a dose of nutmeg and before dinner in order to fortify himself he drank a glass of sack [white wine] - a practice that he recommended to his patients. Afterward he continued on his rounds and before bed drank "my old favorite Liquor, which encouraged Sleep, and an easier Breathing through Pores all Night." Perhaps Dr. Hodges was correct; after all, he survived the Great Plague and lived to write about it.

Many 17th century physicians uncritically relied on anecdotal reports of the efficacy of amulets that often were inscribed with magical or biblical words. The recipe for a popular concoction was guaranteed to protect the wearer. It had been devised by the 16th century French alchemist Paracelsus and called for eighteen desiccated and pulverized toads compounded with specified quantities of the first menstrual blood of young maidens, arsenic, roots, pearls, corals and emeralds. Where did they find all the ingredients? These were mixed to form a paste and shaped into small cakes imprinted with the seals of a serpent and a scorpion. The preparation had to be fabricated at the proper phase of the moon, was enclosed in a metal cylinder that was hung from the neck by a silk ribbon and worn near the heart.

On the Continent there were two more large outbreaks in Vienna (1679) and Marseilles (1720) before the scourge retreated eastward and died out; eventually becoming more a disease of rodents than of men. Presumably disappearance of epidemic plague can't be attributed to strange remedies but to advances in medical science. In our own time plague is considered to be a bacterial disease of rats and bats which when transmitted to man is easily treated with antibiotics. Even today sporadic cases of plague occasionally are reported in the United States but I'm not aware that powdered toad is being prescribed. Perhaps our enlightened president might consider that to be an "interesting" option. After all, it couldn't hurt, could it?

9

QUARANTINE

During the Middle Ages, isolating the sick was thought to be the only effective way of halting periodic epidemics. (It still is.) Ports were understood to be prime entry points and the word "quarantine" was derived from a forty day isolation period that was required of ships entering Venice. During the 15th century the municipality opened its first maritime station (*lazaretto*) for contagious diseases on small off-shore islands, but the concept may have originated with Hippocrates who used 45 days to separate acute from chronic diseases. Within that period of time plague victims either were dead or recovered without having spread their contagion to others.

In America quarantine to combat contagious disease had a long and contentious history. At the beginning of the 19th century, scourges from smallpox and yellow fever had declined, largely as a result of urbanization and crowded tenement life, but they were replaced as a public menace by cholera – indeed, the period between 1832 and 1866 has been described as "the cholera years." Like with bubonic plague, cholera struck suddenly, could kill quickly and there was no effective treatment. It was terrifying.

During a severe outbreak in 1832, New York City's Board of Health assured the public that existing statutes were "full and ample to meet every emergency" and that it had the authority to "exercise all powers as in their judgment the circumstances of the case and the public good shall require." In Malvern, Pennsylvania that same year 57 recently arrived Irish railroad workers died of cholera. Cramped living conditions helped to spread the disease rapidly through the crew and those who tried to seek aid from the local community were shunned. Fear of epidemic cholera along with rising anti-Irish sentiment in the wake of increased immigration created a situation in which these laborers were forced to suffer without any medical relief. It was as if they were a race apart. The men who died in Malvern were hastily buried in a mass grave along the tracks on which they had labored.

That same year epidemic cholera consumed my current hometown Piermont, NY where a community of Irish railroad workers lived in filthy shanties beside the polluted Hudson River. A local reporter bitterly criticized the wealthy class who in his judgment had distanced themselves from the poor victims: "They never enter the cabin of the afflicted lest their garments should be soiled, or their reputation in certain circles depreciated. They can scarcely pass within a hundred yards of the abode of pestilence and poverty without turning up their dainty nose."

Few physicians believed that cholera was contagious; its cause lay in the atmosphere. It was another two decades before they were proved wrong, that it was the water. Prevailing medical opinion opposed quarantine thinking it would serve merely to "flatter vulgar prejudices," and "embarrass with unnecessary restrictions, the commerce and industry of the country." Some insisted that quarantines were "the engines of oppression, despotism and bureaucracy." One physician declared that they were the result of "yielding by the thinking part of the community to the irrational fears of the panic-stricken multitude: Some future historian will record our folly and credulity in the same chapter of events as Salem witchcraft, divining rods, and animal magnetism."

For government not to have enforced quarantines would have been political suicide and, despite the scorn of the medical establishment, a quarantine was established for coastal cities, lake ports and river towns. This strained local budgets for towns which sometimes had to provide for hundreds of quarantined immigrants. When it became evident that quarantine was relatively ineffective as a preventative, cholera "hospitals" were established for the impoverished sick. Because suitable facilities were non-existent, taverns, churches and public schools were pressed into service; to be sure, some argued that the "respectable" poor could be safely treated in their homes rather than in these "slaughterhouses." Nurses were almost impossible to find – it was dirty, dangerous work and, according to one observer, offers of exorbitant salaries attracted only "mercenaries who appear to possess as little sympathy or humanity as the walls."

Every summer from 1850 to 1853 sporadic cases of cholera occurred in Newark, New Jersey but were hidden from the public to avoid unnecessary panic. But by the first week of July 1854 when the disease reached epidemic proportions, many believed that the cause was "Divine Judgment" and the Governor ordered a day of fasting and prayer. A local newspaper reassured its readers that ninety percent of fatalities were those whose "constitutions had previously been injured by intemperate habits." However it soon became apparent that even a man of "regular habits" could be cut down while "the sot that wallowed in the mire of intoxication" often escaped. Immigrants were scapegoated and those who could afford to fled the city. By the time that the last outbreak of cholera in Newark occurred in June, 1866, sanitary cordons were erected around the stricken, homes were vacated and bedding, clothing and personal effects disinfected or destroyed. Only twenty cases developed, and the Board of Health was credited with having prevented an epidemic.

Cholera outbreaks notwithstanding, quarantine of incoming ships as a public health device embroiled New Jersey and New York in a series of disputes through much of the last half of the 19th century. Dr. Ezra M. Hunt, the chairman of New Jersey's Sanitary Commission which advised the Governor and the general public, insisted that moral suasion was ineffective and that only "the strong arm of the law" could properly "turn out, clean out and purify and disinfect, and, if need be, quarantine." During the 1860's and 1870, application of quarantine measures for sick persons frequently involved disputes between sanitarians, who were concerned with clean air, water purification and sewage removal and "anti-contagionists" who argued that once disease had arrived, quarantine was too late.

The germ theory of disease changed much of this. Starting with Newark's Sanitary Code of 1888, physicians were requested to report contagious diseases to the Board of Health which could require isolation of the patient if they thought it necessary. At the end of the century the nurse attending patients in the isolation ward of the Orange Memorial Hospital was not permitted to write letters and could read only such books as could later be burned. The Morristown Board of Health issued a circular which required that any child under 16 years of age who came into town (unless just passing through) was to be placed under quarantine for at least two weeks and inspectors were to go through town daily to seek new arrivals.

By the 1890's most physicians understood that cholera was caused by a water-born bacterium, but the popular perception of the disease as a certain agent of death persisted.

When cholera raged again in New York City in 1892, the Health Department issued frequent bulletins to allay the public's fear. Newspapers and magazines devoted entire issues to covering the epidemic, but the arrival of horse-drawn ambulances, with teams of physicians, sanitary inspectors and policemen at any home where there was a suspicious case of diarrhea was disconcerting.

The eminent bacteriologist William Henry Welch of Johns Hopkins was consulted by William Jenkins, the chief of New York's quarantine station. Welch strongly opposed quarantine and enforced isolation of immigrants and advised the local authorities to cooperate with federal guidelines. Although Jenkins publicly insisted that he was following the consultant's advice, he did the exact opposite. This so enraged Dr. Welch that he described this treachery as "a spectacle of inhumanity without parallel in civilized lands in modern times."

One senator who favored restricting immigration argued that "permitting steamships to enter our ports would overtax all resources and distress our whole people…If we allow immigration we are largely at the mercy of foreigners. If we suspend it our lives are in our own hands. In suspension [of immigration] alone is there any certainty of safety." President Benjamin Harrison got into the act by endorsing a public health circular which established quarantine restrictions on immigration as a means of preventing cholera's entrance into the United States. The circular characterized entering European immigrants as a menace to the public health. Federal law ordered a twenty day quarantine on all potentially infected ships and passengers on these "pest ships" were to be placed in "stations" on tiny off-shore islands. New York City's Tammany-controlled politicians challenged the legality of federal intrusion on their turf although the act stipulated that federal regulations could not conflict with sanitary laws of any state or municipal authorities."

Confrontation between federal and state authorities, panic fanned by incessant media coverage, fluctuating guidelines, appeals for public policy to be guided by science and not by fear – all of these characterized 19th century outbreaks of infectious diseases. In 2014, a nurse just returned from six weeks treating patients in Liberia, wrote to the *Times*, "I have been incredulous, shocked and…angry at the fearful, panicked and, yes, cowardly behavior of the American politicians and public. America needs to get a grip."

Because I originally wrote this essay in 2014 during the Ebola outbreak in West Africa, I suggest that now you re-read the last paragraph and ask yourself what, if anything, has changed?

10
STIMULATE THE PHAGOCYTES

Someone recently observed, "These days we're all immunologists." He exaggerated but it's true that every day over our morning coffee we're bombarded by a bewildering glossary of biologic terms: SARS and MERS, IgG and IgM, chloroquine and remdesivir. What's going on? COVID-19 of course! Or more precisely, SARS-CoV-2. However, the "first-responders" being cheered for going to work are not the only heroes nor the first. The biologic first responders are the B and T lymphocytes that silently work in tandem to mount an immune response against invading pathogens. Normally they interact in a veritable pas-de-deux, the Bs producing antibodies, the Ts scavenging cellular debris.

I read that a small retrospective study from China has reported that many COVID-19 patients have remarkably low T-cell counts in their blood and preliminary trials with tocilizumab (Roche's arthritis drug Actemra) to treat this condition have been impressive. Apparently the mechanism of this drug's action involves *stimulating* depleted T cells and that sounded familiar to me. Let me explain why.

George Bernard Shaw's satiric play *The Doctor's Dilemma*, first staged in London in 1906, concerned the conflicts between the demands of the business side of private practice and the moral obligations of the profession. In one memorable scene, a group of doctors gather to congratulate their colleague Dr. Colenso Ridgeon who has just been knighted for his success in treating tubercular patients. His method was to inoculate them with an injectable anti-toxin, thereby "stimulating the phagocytes." As they engage in shop talk. Ridgeon declares that the key to successful phagocytosis is to "butter the disease germs with opsonin to make your white blood corpuscles eat them."

The gastrointestinal metaphor was apt because the word opsonin is derived from the Greek opsōneîn, meaning to prepare for eating. Opsonins aid the immune system in a number of ways. In a healthy individual, they mark dead and dying cells for clearance by macrophages and neutrophils, activate complement proteins, and target cells for destruction through the action of natural killer cells. To continue the metaphor, opsonin causes the phagocyte to relish the tasty invader. What follows next is some of G.B. Shaw's dialogue:

> Sir Patrick Cullen (a much older physician):*"That's not new. I've heard the notion of white corpuscles…what's his name, Metchnikoff calls them….?"*

> Ridgeon*: "Phagocytes."*

> Sir Patrick: *"Aye phagocytes: yes, yes, yes. Well I heard this theory that the phagocytes eat up the disease germs years ago: long before you came into fashion. Besides they don't always eat them….I've tried these modern inoculations a bit myself. I've killed people with them; and I've cured people with them; but I gave them up because I never could tell which I was going to do.*

> Ridgeon: *"They [get better] when you butter them with opsonin….What it comes to in practice is this. The phagocytes won't eat the microbes unless the microbes are nicely buttered for them. Well, the patient manufactures the butter for himself all right; but my discovery is that the manufacture of that butter, which I call opsonin, goes on in the system by ups and downs - Nature always being*

rhythmical, you know. What the inoculation does is to stimulate the ups or downs as the case may be.....Everything depends on your inoculating at the right moment. Inoculate when your patient is in the negative phase, the downgrade, and you kill: inoculate when the patient is in the positive phase, up-grade, and you cure."

In Shaw's play, Sir Colenso Ridgeon's stated that by sending "a drop of blood" to the hospital laboratory, he could establish a numerical "opsonin index" that indicated when it was safe to inoculate: "That's my discovery: the most important that has been made since Harvey discovered the circulation of blood. My tuberculosis patients don't die now." As Shaw's doctors continued to gossip, the authoritative Sir Ralph Bloomfield Bonington spoke up. (GBS notes: "He is known in the medical world as B.B.; and the envy roused by his success in practice is softened by the conviction that he is scientifically considered a colossal humbug."):

B.B.:*There is at bottom only one genuinely scientific treatment for all diseases, and that is to stimulate the phagocytes. Stimulate the phagocytes. Drugs are a delusion. Find the germ of the disease; prepare from it a suitable anti-toxin; inject it three times a day quarter of an hour before meals; and what is the result? The phagocytes are stimulated; they devour the disease' and the patient recovers - unless, of course, he's too far gone....*

Everything is dangerous unless you take it at the right time. An apple at breakfast does you good: an apple at bedtime upsets you for a week. There are only two rules for antitoxins. First, don't be afraid of them: second, inject them a quarter of an hour before meals, three times a day.

Ridgeon: (appalled) *Great heavens, B.B., no, no, no.*

George Bernard Shaw was a severe critic of medical hypocrisy and unfairness. Also he was well versed in contemporary science and this was the basis for *The Doctor's Dilemma*. In 1911 Shaw added a lengthy preface to his play in which he credited the biologist Sir Almroth Wright as being the first to describe "the perils" of inoculation, that injection of strong 'vaccines' at the wrong moment, might reinforce the disease instead of stimulating resistance to it. [Note: A historian once described Almroth Wright as "a romantic who only accepted those pieces of science that suited him."] Shaw continues:

> *Sir Almroth Wright, following up one of Metchnikoff's most suggestive biological romances, discovered [in 1902] that the white corpuscles or phagocytes which attack and devour the disease germs appetizingly for them with a natural sauce which Sir Almroth named opsonin, and that our production of this condiment continually rises and falls rhythmically from negligibility to the highest efficiency... By the time this preface is in print...opsonin may have gone the way of phlogiston.*

In 1888, Louis Pasteur invited the Russian-born scientist Elie Metchnikoff to join the Pasteur Institute in Paris. While there he discovered the process of phagocytosis that demonstrated how specific white cells can break down harmful bacteria in the body. Metchnikoff reasoned that inflammation was merely a cellular response to an external agent, a body's curative reaction. What he called phagocytes included many types of white blood cells (e.g. neutrophils, monocytes, macrophages, mast cells) and also he coined the term opsonin for an antibody which binds to foreign microorganisms making them more susceptible to digestion by white cells. Elie Metchnikoff and the German chemist Paul Ehrlich shared the Nobel Prize in Physiology or Medicine in 1908 "in recognition of their work on immunity." Curiously, today each of them is remembered for something else.

Metchnikoff is regarded as the grandfather of modern probiotics. It was he who observed that the regular consumption of lactobacilli in fermented dairy products, such as yogurt, was associated with enhanced health and longevity in Bulgarian peasants. He theorized that these healthy bacteria helped digestion and improved the phagocytic capability of white blood cells. To test the benefits of consuming lactobacilli, he drank sour milk every day until he died at the ripe age of 71 years in 1916.

One year after sharing the Nobel Prize with Metchnikoff, Paul Ehrlich and his team of researchers developed an arsenic based compound (arsphenamine) that was the first effective agent to treat syphilis. Along with his research team, Ehrlich experimented with hundreds of compounds until finally succeeding on their 606th attempt. The injected drug that came to market in 1910 was called Salvarsan and was used until penicillin came along in the 1940s. It was the first modern chemotherapeutic agent, sometimes referred to as "the magic bullet" or simply as "606."

That returns us to the present because economic, societal and political considerations notwithstanding, science can't be rushed. Currently more than 100 laboratories throughout the world are racing to find a vaccine and anti-viral drugs that are effective against COVID-19. Naturally, to the winners will belong tremendous spoils and because successful activation of T lymphocytes is critical to the immune system's ability to clear infections, research increasingly is focusing on them. To use current media parlance, T cells are "essential workers."

Earlier I mentioned a retrospective study from China which found that 76 percent of COVID-19 patients had remarkably low T-cell counts in their blood - especially those being treated in intensive care. The investigators suggested that the virus triggers an overproduction of pro-inflammatory cytokines which in turn contribute to exhaustion and depletion of T cells. As patients gradually recovered, their T cell counts rose while cytokine levels dramatically declined. Based on these findings, the research team concluded that it's the storm itself that promotes dysfunction or even death of these critical cells.

Various monoclonal antibodies currently are being studied in order to prevent or control potentially life-threatening cytokine storms by blocking overproduction of interleukins derived from B cells. But as one Chinese investigator has suggested, we should pay more attention to T cell counts and their function especially for those patients with low T lymphocyte counts. Treating potentially lethal cytokine storms by boosting T-cells seems to make sense and I suspect that were Shaw's character Colenso Ridgeon around today, he would agree. Moreover, I imagine that he would advise modern physicians to STIMULATE THE PHAGOCYTES! And if so, he might have been correct.

11
VACCINATION

Of paramount concern during this pandemic has been development of a safe and effective vaccine. Currently more than one hundred pharmaceutical companies are vying to win the global competition for the Covid-19 virus and the lucrative manufacturing and distribution contracts that will follow. That got me thinking about the long history of vaccinations.

Inhalation or introduction through the skin of material from fresh small pox lesions was practiced in China during the 10th century and perhaps as early as 1000 BC in India. Long before Edward Jenner found that cowpox conferred immunity, it was common knowledge that survivors of smallpox became immune to recurrence and inoculation (or "variolation") by lancet of pus from a sick to a healthy person could prevent them from contracting a serious case. This was practiced throughout the world. In the Caucasus where the women were legendary beauties, girls were inoculated early lest their fair skin be marred if later they were deemed to be candidates for the Ottoman sultan's harem. When Lady Montagu, the wife of the English ambassador to Turkey, whose own face was disfigured by smallpox, arrived in Istanbul and learned of the local custom, she had her children inoculated and when she returned home in 1718 was credited with introducing the method of variolation in England.

In Colonial America George Washington, his own face permanently marked by a childhood case of the pox, feared that the epidemic's "calamitous consequences" would be more deadly than "the sword of the enemy." He had a difficult choice to make for although mass inoculation was the preferred course, what would happen if the British learned that most of the Continentals were recuperating and too weak to fight? After much agonizing, the decision was made to inoculate and the army was able to pull it off without letting the enemy know their battle readiness - it was the first government mandated immunization program. In 1788 Benjamin Franklin wrote the following:

> *In 1736 I lost one of my sons, a fine boy of four years old, by the small pox taken in the common way. I long regretted bitterly, and still regret, that I had not given to him by inoculation. This I mention for the sake of parents who omit this operation on the supposition that they never should forgive themselves if a child died under it; my example showing that the regret may be the same either way, and that, therefore, the safer should be chosen.*

Currently I live in Rockland County, New York which once was a hotbed of vaccine production. That was thanks to the efforts of four remarkable men and what follows next are brief biographies of these pioneers: Paul Gibier, Ernst Lederle, Herold Cox and Hilary Koprowski.

Paul Gibier (1851-1900) was a French-born doctor and bacteriologist who founded the New York Pasteur Institute, a pioneering research laboratory that was concerned with developing vaccines and anti-toxins. As a young man he had served in the French cavalry in Africa before attending the University of Paris where in 1884 he obtained a degree in medicine. His doctoral thesis concerned rabies in animals and soon after graduation, the French government sent him to Spain to study cholera and then on to Havana to study yellow fever. For his work he was awarded a gold medal and was made a Chevalier of the Legion of Honour.

While studying for a short time with Louis Pasteur in Paris, Gibier became fascinated with what he called "spiritism" or "psychism" and was intrigued by the exploits of a woman known by the pseudonym "Mrs. Salmon." Actually she was Carrie Sawyer, a well-known illusionist, psychic and probable fraud. Dr. Gibier was impressed with her seances that seemed to support his own belief that intelligence exists separate from the body and confirmed the concept of immortality. He formed a circle of like-minded people and published a book in which he discussed mediums, North American Indians and Hindu Fakirs and explored hypnotism, telepathy, etc. Not surprisingly, there were skeptics and critics and he felt obliged to immigrate to America's more receptive soil.

In 1890, presumably with his mentor's approval, Gibier established at 313 West 23rd Street in Manhattan what he called the Pasteur Institute for inoculation of people who'd been bitten by rabid animals. In the clinic's first year 828 people were seen of whom 643 were found to not have rabies, but 185 were inoculated with the revolutionary Pasteur vaccine and none died. Dr. Gibier was an impresario who was able to win public interest and gain financial and social support for his research and development institute which some believe lay the foundation for the modern bio-medical industry. He may have originated the idea of serotherapy in order to treat cancer suggesting to the Paris Academy of Sciences "to infuse to an animal, the juice of human tumor and to use the blood or the serum of this animal to infuse in the human harboring this tumor." He improvised new methods of culturing microbes and producing sera and antitoxins and the institute on Central Park West was the first in the United States to produce a diphtheria antitoxin.

Dr. Gibier became a member of the New York Academy of Medicine and edited a quarterly journal that not only included results of his and his colleagues work, but also translations of foreign medical articles, reports on rabies treatments and advertisements for medical devices and products for practitioners. Gibier boldly advanced the view that the medical "priest" should lead a movement away from "sentimental" toward "scientific religion." A prolific writer, he argued that only the doctor could properly diagnose such "diseases" as socialism and anarchy, and that with his knowledge of genetics he could "contribute to the purification of the race" through marriage counseling.

Several months after his Institute opened in 1893, Gibier explained in a feature article in the *New York Times* how frantic patients were flocking to his clinic from all over the country and Canada. Rabies treatment required more than a dozen daily injections over about three weeks and for "poor patients" their home cities usually paid travel and housing expenses. Those who could not afford to pay were treated free. Another article about the Institute headlined "The Defenders of the Human Body and Their Foes. What Is Being Done at the New York Pasteur Institute to Enlarge Our Knowledge of Health and Disease."

Preparation of antitoxins took two months and required large amounts of serum. Mr. C.G. West of Greenwich Connecticut who owned stables in New York, whose son was twice treated by Gibier (once for diphtheria, once for hydrophobia) was so grateful that he donated a prize-winning brood mare and the use of sixty stalls for horses to be inoculated both for test purposes and preparation of antiserum. A newspaper account noted that Dr. Gidier already had forty horses in another stable and because he also had numerous dogs, sheep and guinea pigs to be sacrificed as "martyrs to science," clearly there was a need for farmland. Rockland County beckoned.

In 1895 Dr. Gibier bought a 183 acres farm on the Nyack Turnpike, on the outskirts of Suffern, about 30 miles northwest of New York City. There he set up a "Pasteur Farm" where he bred animals in order to have sufficient serum available for production of vaccines and anti-toxins. A local newspaper article at the time described the doctor as "a man of magnificent physique who never used tobacco or stimulants." A large wood and stone frame sanitorium was built on the grounds to care for tubercular patients. In addition to the conventional fresh air and rest treatment they received injections of antitoxins to TB as well as to streptococcus and staphylococcus - the prices varied from 25 cents to five dollars a shot; the price for a room varied between $12 and $25 per week.

Paul Gibier maintained contact with his medium "Mrs. Salmon" (Carrie M. Sawyer) and for ten years conducted experiments with her both in his New York laboratory and at his country home. He planned to take her to England, France and Egypt but his plans were cut short when he was killed in a tragic accident. As he and his sister-in-law rode on his Suffern estate, the horse pulling his carriage was spooked by a gun shot, ran away and the carriage overturned. The 50 year old doctor was thrown out and died a few hours later from a skull fracture. His wife claimed that the night before the accident, he'd told her of a dream he'd just had that predicted that he would die after being thrown from his buggy. He had laughed at her fears. The spiritualist journal *Banner of Light* lamented that the movement had lost one of its truest friends.

Another New York City experimenter who needed lots of pasture land for his "animal martyrs" was chemist **Ernst Lederle** (1865 -1921) who in 1906 bought an 88 acre dairy farm in Pearl River for his Lederle Antitoxin Laboratories. Lederle was born on Staten Island in 1865, was employed by New York City in 1889 as a milk inspector and assistant chemist. When smallpox broke out in the city's tenements in 1900, Lederle, by now the city's chief chemist, was sent to Europe to learn new methods of prevention and treatment. When another epidemic broke out two years later, Lederle was appointed the city's Commissioner of Health and employed an emergency force of some 200 vaccinators to work the tenements and places of business, accompanied by policemen. More than 800,000 people were vaccinated within six months - everyone within a two block radius of every reported case. All told in 1901 there had been 1,198 cases of small pox in New York City with 410 deaths; after Lederle's campaign in 1902 there were 309 deaths and the next year only four.

As Health Commissioner Ernst Lederle promoted pasteurization laws against raw milk which might cause tuberculosis and achieved some fame by organizing campaigns for "certified" milk. He heard complaints about such things as barking dogs, smoke and poor ventilation in streetcars, dead animals on the streets and the bad manners of hospital attendants. He opened dental clinics for school children, started venereal disease clinics and fought epidemics of polio and typhoid and banned the common drinking cup. In 1910, out of sympathy for the plight of "Typhoid Mary", Lederle released her from quarantine on North Brother Island in the East River where the city maintained an isolation hospital. Three years later Mary broke her promise to Lederle that she would never work as a cook again and resumed her profession under an assumed name so there was another outbreak of typhoid. She was recommitted to spend the rest of her life on the island - a total of twenty-six years in quarantine!

Ernst Lederle fell out of favor with the Tammany machine and in 1903 was replaced, but wasting no time, he formed Lederle Laboratories for "chemical, bacteriological and sanitary investigations and analysis" and soon decided that there was a good business opportunity in producing improved diphtheria antitoxin. In order to increase supply Lederle needed horse serum - plenty of it, so in 1906 he purchased the farm in Pearl River that would provide plenty of pasture land for his herd. A robust horse named Jumbo gave a prodigious total of 450 gallons of blood over thirteen years before being retired, presumably depleted. Later on horse serum was replaced by rabbit serum, earning Pearl River the title "Rabbit City." Ernst Lederle's second stint as Health Commissioner ended in 1914, just four years before the Spanish Flu pandemic. In 1921, only three weeks after his wife died, he succumbed to septicemia in a sanitarium in Goshen, N.Y.

Herald Cox (1907-1986) began at the Rockefeller Institute in 1932 and developed vaccines against equine encephalitis. The U.S. Public Health Service sent him to Montana to discover a cure for Rocky Mountain Spotted Fever, was infected by the deadly bacterium but was saved only because he self-administered his own vaccine. He was made principal bacteriologist of the Public Health Service at age 33, the youngest ever to hold the top scientific post. In 1942 Cox began working at Lederle and where he did basic research on epidemic typhus that allowed the company to produce over 90,000 vaccine doses daily so that not a single death was reported among millions of immunized troops neither World War II or Korea.

Next Cox turned to developing an attenuated live vaccine against polio and enlisted a recently arrived young scientist by the name of **Hilary Koprowski** for the project. Dr. Cox went on to receive many prestigious awards and later spent four years as director of cancer research at Roswell Park Memorial Institute in Buffalo. Koprowski fled his native Poland in 1939 and settled in Brazil where he took a research position funded by the Rockefeller Foundation studying yellow fever vaccine. But when offered a position at Lederle in Pearl River he accepted and upon arrival was put to work on a rabies vaccine.

Two years later, medical director Cox, assigned Koprowski to the polio project studying monkeys, mice and rats. By 1948 his work progressed to the point that he and his chief assistant were emboldened to swallow a vile-tasting blend of spinal cord and brain taken from an infected rat. As adults, they already had antibodies against polio but the question was whether their live but weakened virus was safe. It was and they survived.

At about that same time, the medical director at nearby Letchworth Village, Dr. George Jervis, feared that they faced a polio epidemic because the virus gets transmitted from feces to hand and mouth and some of the retarded boys at Letchworth were fond of throwing feces at each other. Jervis knew that scientists at Lederle were working on a live oral polio vaccine and were eager to test it in humans. The first guinea pig was a six year old boy who in 1950 was given the vaccine to drink in some chocolate milk. Within two weeks he developed antibodies and didn't get sick. Nineteen more presumably "volunteer" children followed with the same result. When Hilary Koprowski presented his data at a major meeting, Jonas Salk objected to the fact that the initial research involved human beings. Salk's own work involved prisoners and mentally retarded inmates of an institution in Pennsylvania while field trials of Sabin's vaccine had been conducted on millions of people in Russia.

That's how research was done during the 1940s and 50s. When the Salk vaccine was introduced in 1955 it used a killed virus although effective and safe needed to be injected three times. At the same time Albert Sabin copied the Lederle technique that used an oral attenuated live virus but his method required giving three separate doses six weeks apart, each for one of the three strains of polio virus. After the first tests in Pearl River, Cox and Koprowski's vaccine was safely administered in

1958 to 250,000 individuals in the Belgian Congo and that same year in a mass immunization program in Dade County, Florida.

Although the work of these four virologists reduced the untold suffering of children and young adults worldwide, it was Jonas Salk and Albert Sabin who received most of the glory and financial report from the March of Dimes. Nevertheless Lederle's single dose trivalent oral vaccine would surpass both Salk's injectable killed virus vaccine and Sabin's monovalent oral live vaccine that was introduced in stages in the early 1960s. In 1963 Lederle was the first company to be licensed to produce all three strains In a single oral preparation that was easier to administer and provided longer lasting immunity. In later years a sign on Route 303 outside the Lederle plant read "Welcome to Pearl River, Polio Vaccine Capitol of the World.

Hilary Koprowski (1916 - 2013) was a multi-talented scientist, but was headstrong with a sometimes abrasive personality. In 1957 he left Lederle and took over a moribund vaccine producer in Philadelphia and transformed Wistar, into a leader in biology, virology, immunology, cancer research, and aging. In the 1970s, scientists at the Institute were among the first to develop antiviral and antitumor cell monoclonal antibodies and in the early 1980s, Wistar became a leader in studies of human cancer genetics.

Hilary Koprowski was highly cultured, a patron of the arts and a superb pianist. A colleague recalled him as "a special person…one of the pioneers in vaccine development [who played] a key role in protecting our population against the ravages of virus diseases." Hilary Koprowski became wealthy and continued his research into his 90s, outliving his rivals Salk and Sabin in age but not in fame.

In due time Lederle Laboratories expanded its product line to include numerous vaccines, vitamins, sulfa drugs and antibiotics and at its peak more than 3,000 people worked in Pearl River. Today the plant is owned by Pfizer whose chief priority is developing a vaccine against Covid-19. By mid-July the Federal government was prepared to sign a nearly two billion dollar contract for the company to produce 600 million doses of the still-unfinished vaccine should it prove to be safe and effective in a phase 3 trial.

12
EPIDEMIOLOGY

Everyone has heard the name Noah Webster, but few know much about the man or his work other than his famous dictionary. But that wasn't his only literary work and among his various contributions was a two volume book published in 1799 titled *A Brief History of Epidemic and Pestilential Diseases with the Principal Phenomena of the Physical World, Which precede and Accompany Them and Observations Deduced From the Facts Stated.* Although little remembered today, during the 19th century this book was a standard text in American medical schools. William Osler in 1902 called it "the most important medical work written in this country by a layman." Pathologist Aldred.S. Warthin (1923) suggested that the book "might well entitle Webster to be designated 'the father of American epidemiology.'"

Noah Webster was *not* a man of few words. His dictionary attested to that; indeed this "brief" history of epidemic and pestilential diseases totaled 709 pages! The title page noted that he was "Author of Dissertations on the English Language and several other Works." But why did this obsessive wordsmith spend three years writing a history of diseases about which he had no more than a layman's knowledge? Before I attempt to answer that question, a brief review of salient features of his biography may be useful.

Born in West Hartford, Connecticut in 1758, Noah graduated from Yale in 1778. He passed the bar examination but finding himself unable to find work as a lawyer, he opened a private school and wrote a series of educational books. In 1793, Alexander Hamilton recruited Webster to move to New York City where he became an editor for a Federalist Party newspaper. He published newspaper articles, political essays, and textbooks but in 1798 he returned to Connecticut. Eight years later Webster published his first dictionary, *A Compendious Dictionary of the English Language*. The following year, he began work on the more comprehensive version that we know.

From 1812 to 1822, Webster and his family lived in Amherst, Massachusetts where he was one of the founders of what became Amherst College. Living largely off the income from his published schoolbooks, Webster served in the Massachusetts legislature and continued work on his expanded dictionary that finally was published in 1828. While working on a second volume he died in 1843 at age 85, and the rights to the dictionary were acquired by George and Charles Merriam. Some have called Noah Webster the "Father of American Scholarship and Education" but what does any of this have to do with epidemiology? I'll let the great man speak for himself and what follows next is extracted from his Introduction to Volume One.

> *A publication on the subject of diseases from the pen of a man who has never before turned his attention to medical science or to chemistry is a circumstance, which, if it does not require an apology, demands at least an explanation….*

> *The prevalence of the catarrh, commonly called influenza, in the years 1789 and 90, fully awakened my curiosity on the subject of epidemic diseases. A journey which I made in October 1789 from Hartford to Boston, and another in March 1790 from Hartford to Albany, led me to observe the progressiveness of that disease, with its other phenomena….A slight attack which my own children suffered, in May following, together with a similar attack*

of many other children in Hartford, and its more violent effects some months after, convinced me that the epidemic was progressive in malignancy, as well as in regard to place.

Had no other epidemic appeared, my curiosity would probably have subsided and been extinguished. The malignant fever in New York in 1791 had excited alarm in that city and was a subject of notice in Hartford where I then resided, but no idea had been conceived, that it was connected with a pestilential state of the air, in the United States, which was afterwards to produce more ferocious and general calamities.

In autumn of 1793 however that pestilential state of air arrived to its crisis in Philadelphia, where the mortality occasioned by the yellow fever spread destruction and dismay from August to November. The fatality of the disease spread consternation thro the United States and excited apprehensions in Europe…No American citizen could be indifferent to the prevalence of this disease in his own country. Still it was conceived that the distemper might have been produced from imported infection and that a more rigid execution of the laws relating to quarantine might prevent a repetition of the calamity.

Tranquility was of short duration. The appearance of the same disease in New Haven in 1794, and in New York, Baltimore and Norfolk in 1795, revived my curiosity, with double zeal to search out the causes of these phenomena, so unusual in this country. The facts which had come to my knowledge relating to the origin and propagation of this disease led me to suspect the common theory of infection to be ill-founded.

> *But as a preliminary to all other enquiries, it appeared*
> *necessary to settle the controversy relative to the imported*
> *or domestic sources of the distemper for without a decision*
> *of this question, legislative and police regulations for*
> *preventing a return of the evil, or mitigating its severity,*
> *would probably be fruitless. The question appeared to be*
> *extremely important and the differences of opinion on the*
> *subject among medical gentlemen seemed to preclude the*
> *possibility of a decision among them that would silence*
> *doubts in the public mind.*

The remainder of the two volumes was devoted to a meticulous description of plagues and pestilences from ancient times to his own. Webster was skeptical of conventional medical wisdom and his emphasis always was on the association of diseases with climatologic or celestial events.

Noah Webster's skepticism of received wisdom and his zeal to seek answers for himself was admirable. He insisted that facts are "the only genuine source of knowledge" but his conclusion that "visible and remarkable" phenomena were the culprit was seriously flawed. Of course, he lived nearly a century before the advent of germ theory. Webster began his research by writing to physicians and scholars throughout the country, but their understanding of pathophysiology was as mistaken as his own. The most famous of them all, Philadelphia's Benjamin Rush, strove to eliminate bad humors by aggressively "bleeding, blistering, purging and puking." Historians often refer to that approach as "heroic medicine" but the true heroes were Rush's patients whose teeth fell out from mercury toxicity and suffered more from the treatment than the disease.

Webster haunted libraries in New York, Philadelphia and Boston and the result of all his labors was a voluminous (not "brief") history of plagues and pestilences from earliest times until his own. What Noah Webster called his "general pestilential principle" was that epidemic diseases frequently resulted from extremes of weather and/or natural occurrences as floods and fires, earthquakes and volcanic eruptions and, especially, passing meteors and comets. Such natural events caused fetid air or miasma (from a Latin word meaning noxious vapors) which, in turn, caused illness. "Infection is capable of all degrees of activity and force, from a slight impurity of air, which affects no person in health, to that virulent state of air which will produce vomiting in a person suddenly exposed to it."

Even as Noah Webster was developing his general theory, most of his contemporaries suspected that periodic plagues were brought to American shores by sea travelers from afar. Among those who held such a view was Ezra Stiles, president of Yale, who documented the fevers and plagues that swept through New Haven during his tenure (1778-1795) in a "Literary Diary". During an outbreak of scarlet fever in 1794, about two thirds of the students were stricken and classes were suspended for nearly two months. Those who remained in town were offered tutors but three months after the fever finally abated another plague swept through New Haven.

At the end of 1794 President Stiles calculated the year's grim total: out of a student population of about 3,500, 50 died of scarlet fever, 63 of yellow fever and 70 either of other sicknesses or had "died at sea." Medical historian George Rosen vividly described Webster's "sally into the arena of medical disputation": "Whether Webster is depicted as a swashbuckling scholar making a strike into foreign territory or as an absentminded professor who lost his way and wandered into strange fields, a somewhat perplexed attitude is implied in both." Perplexing seems an apt description. Exasperating might be another.

Why should we now take time to recall this sincere but futile attempt by a misinformed non-scientist to make sense of the still undiscovered world of microbes? It's because there's an uncanny similarity to current events. During these Covid days, scientists exhort us to rely on proven facts rather than on half-baked ideas and wishful thinking. A caveat is that "facts" sometimes can deceive and, alas, that was the fatal flaw in Noah Webster's attempt to understand the mystery of epidemics and pestilences. But good try Noah!

13

HAND WASHING

Sing *Happy Birthday* twice - or count slowly to twenty - and scrub, scrub, scrub! We've become a nation of compulsive hand washers, just like Lady MacBeth, but it wasn't always so. Before Pasteur and Koch ushered in germ theory, cleanliness was considered unmanly by self-respecting physicians. When did things change?

If you thought that Ignaz Semmelweis was the first to insist upon cleanliness to prevent puerperal (childbed) fever you'd be wrong. The laurels should go to Boston's poet-physician Oliver Wendell Holmes Sr. His first paper about transmission of childbed (puerperal) fever was read to the Boston Society for Medical Improvement on February 15, 1843. In "The Contagiousness of Puerperal Fever" (1855) he defended a critique that he'd made two years earlier in which he argued that child-bed fever was related to unclean practices by doctors, nurses and attendants who carried the disease from patient to patient. Holmes was outraged at how medical colleagues were ignoring obvious facts and after one particularly egregious incident, he sarcastically remarked:

> *In view of these facts it does appear a singular coincidence*
> *that one man or woman should have ten, twenty, thirty or*
> *seventy cases of this rare disease following his or her footsteps*
> *with the keenness of a beagle, through the streets and lanes*

*of a crowded city, while the scores that cross the same paths
on the same errands know it only by name.*

O.W. Holmes concluded, "The time has come when the existence of a private pestilence in the sphere of a single physician should be looked upon not as a misfortune, but a crime." This declaration provoked howls of protest, most vociferously by the eminent Philadelphia obstetrician Charles Meigs who dismissed any such suggestion: "Doctors are gentlemen and gentlemen's hands are clean." However, Oliver Wendell Holmes was never one to back down:

> *I am too much in earnest for either humility or vanity, but I do entreat those who hold the keys of life and death to listen to me also for this once. I ask no personal favor; but I beg to be heard on behalf of the women whose lives are at stake until some stronger voice shall plead for them…. In my own family, I had rather that those I esteemed the most should be delivered unaided in a stable, by the manger side, than that they should receive the best help in the finest departments, but exposed to the vapors of this pitiless disease.*

Dr. Holmes closed his fifty page tirade by suggesting "it might be proper to consult the languid survivors, the widowed husbands, and the motherless children."

Four years later Dr. Ignaz Semmelweiss was working in the obstetrics department at the Vienna General Hospital, when he observed that mortality was three times greater on doctors' wards than on midwives' wards. About the same time one of his friends was accidentally cut while performing an autopsy and died. When this doctor's post mortem exam revealed pathology similar to that seen in women dying of puerperal fever Semmelweis made the connection. He deduced that students were transmitting "cadaverous particles" on their hands from the autopsy room to the obstetrics clinic and he established a policy of washing hands with a solution of chlorinated lime, called hypochlorous acid, after performing autopsies and before obstetrical deliveries. Although obstetrical mortality was drastically reduced, Semmelweis was unable to provide an explanation that was satisfactory to his medical colleagues.

> *Puerperal fever is caused by conveyance to the pregnant*
> *of putrid particles derived from living organisms, through*
> *the agency of the examining fingers…Consequently, must*
> *I make my confession that God only knows the number of*
> *women whom I have consigned prematurely to the grave.*

Ridiculed and rejected by the medical community, Semmelweis became agitated and then depressed and four years after his discovery, he was committed to an asylum. Two weeks after admission he was beaten by guards and during the melee cut his finger. Ironically, the champion of asepsis died of sepsis at age 47 from a cut finger.

So although history credited Ignaz Semmelweis for being "the savior of mothers" it really was Oliver Wendell Holmes Sr. who first championed the cause of antisepsis in the delivery room. But despite the work of Holmes and Semmelweis most hospitals continued to practice surgery under unsanitary conditions. Surgeons fondly referred to "the good old surgical stink" and took pride in the stains on their unwashed gowns as a display of their experience. It took another two decades before the antiseptic principles grudgingly adopted in obstetrical delivery rooms began to be applied in surgical suites.

While working at the Glasgow Royal Infirmary, British surgeon Joseph Lister became aware of a recently published paper by Louis Pasteur that described the role of microbes in spoiled milk and wine. At about the same time carbolic acid, derived from coal tar, not only was found to be useful in protecting wood from rotting but also removed unpleasant fecal smells of cattle. Lister reasoned that the same phenomenon could occur in decomposing flesh and began testing the chemical's efficacy when applied directly to wounds.

Operative mortality plummeted and when the results were published in 1867, surgeons were advised to wear clean gloves and wash their hands with carbolic acid (phenol) both before and after operations.

Instruments were washed in the same solution and assistants sprayed the room. But American surgeon Howard Kelly was not impressed and grumbled, "If used in strength sufficient to certainly prevent sepsis, the patient is very often killed along with the germs."

In 1881, German microbiologist Robert Koch found that bacilli thrived in wounds treated with carbolic acid and advocated the use of pressurized steam to sterilize anything that came in contact with the patient, from instruments to surgeon's gowns. Eventually carbolic acid was discarded because of toxicity and supplanted by other antiseptic agents. Although Lister's ideas initially were rejected by colleagues, late in life he received many prestigious honors and was knighted. In 1879 an American doctor developed an alcohol-based formula for a surgical antiseptic and named it in honor of Lord Lister. *Listerine* continues to be used today as a mouthwash. I wonder whether President Trump swallows it.

14

TRIAGE

A recent article in the *New Yorker* (April 20, 2020) described how back in 1985 Gov. Mario Cuomo appointed a multidiscipline Task Force on Life and the Law in order to advise New York State on "ethically tricky" public policy issues. That same year New Jersey Gov. Jim Florio appointed a similar Bioethics Commission of about two dozen people from different backgrounds. I was one of three physician members and the next six years may have been the most stimulating period of my professional career as we commissioners also discussed "ethically tricky" issues and some of our recommendations were incorporated into statutory law.

One thing that we *didn't* consider was triage. Although this subject often comes up in abstract bioethical discussions, it's usually in the context of war and I never expected that some day the issue would arise in my own relatively safe world. Fortunately, as far as I know, so far there haven't been any instances in this country of doctors having to make choices about who gets the last ventilator (or dialysis machine.) Hopefully we'll squeeze by, but I'd like to make a few points concerning the *process* of how such decisions should get made and by whom.

That *New Yorker* article described how recently an ad hoc group that included members of the original New York State Task Force, recently had developed a list of exclusion criteria (e.g. brain injury, severe burns, survivors of recent cardiac arrest, etc.) They proposed that designated groups of doctor/bioethicists should make critical allocation decisions, thereby removing the onus from bedside physicians. Moreover, such decisions would be made according to policy and, although this approach has appeal, it does evoke disturbing memories of Sarah Palin's infamous "death panels."

New York's Department of Health chose not to endorse the ad hoc committee's proposals, but an example of how this might work was provided when New Jersey's Department of Health distributed its own guidelines. They advised all hospitals to create an "acute care triage team" of at least one physician, nurse and administrator to avoid conflict of interest and "minimize moral distress" so that patient's clinicians are not the ones making decisions. Patients would be assigned a score from 1 to 8 based on how likely they are to survive and benefit from intensive care and if the triage team needs a tiebreaker, "higher priority would be given to younger patients, a sick health care worker and others 'critical to the public health response or maintaining societal order.'….[and] If there is still a tie the triage team can use a lottery system." Why not just flip a coin?

Bioethicist Ezekiel Emanuel sometimes writes for the *New York Times* and has been ubiquitous on television. In recent journal articles (*New England Journal of Medicine*, March 28 and May 21) he discussed principles for fair allocation of scarce resources, the intent being to maximize the benefits produced (in this case, by scarce ventilators), treating people equally and giving priority to the worst off. Dr. Emanuel favors establishing "consistent policies that allow life or death decisions to be made while removed from duress at the bedside. That's very good, but more problematic is Dr. Emanuel's suggestion that it's justifiable to remove a patient from a ventilator or an ICU bed in order to provide it to others even without their consent - perhaps even over their objections. He suggests that for patients with similar prognoses, equality should be invoked and operationalized through random allocation, such as a lottery, rather than on a first-come, first-served process.

A basic Jewish tenet is that we all are created in God's image, but that we don't possess absolute dominion over our bodies. It's as if we are only tenants and, therefore, obligated to take care of what doesn't belong to us. According to Jewish tradition we must do everything possible to save life regardless of its quality and that saving one life is equal to saving the world *(pikuah nefesh)*. Whether or not you agree with this, I'm sure that none of us would want rigid bureaucratic policy to devalue certain lives - after all, what about the disabled or mentally challenged? Should they lose their rights to that last ventilator?

History teaches us that the extreme end result of utilitarian thinking could be what occurred in Nazi Germany during the 1930s when what began as sterilization of the "unfit" led to euthanasia - what they called "mercy killing" - with the justification of serving the greater good of the people, the *volk*. Everyone knows what came next: genocide and Holocaust.

15
WHEN IS DEATH?

These COVID days, mortality figures are on everyone's minds, but in much earlier times among occasionally perplexing challenges was how to diagnose when death actually had occurred. Indeed anxiety over being buried alive dates back many centuries. Roman author Pliny the Elder remarked: "Such is the condition of humanity, and so uncertain is men's judgment, that they cannot determine even death itself." The New Testament told of Jesus raising the beggar Lazarus from the dead. (In modern times dozens of cases have been reported of a so-called "Lazarus Syndrome" - spontaneous return of normal heart rhythm after failed attempts at resuscitation.) Maimonides cited much earlier Greek sources that described cases of deep sleep simulating death for prolonged periods up to 72 hours after such causes as asphyxia, ingestion of poisons or intoxicants, insect bites, suddenly eating bread after not tasting it for a long time and coitus after long abstinence.

Lively debate continued for centuries and, in particular, the 19th century was obsessed by reports of inadvertent live burials. Other than holding a feather or a mirror next to the nose, doctors had few means of certifying death except for visible decay and many skeptics about their skill were quick to sensationalize any mistakes. Sometimes bells were tied to a cadaver's limbs that could be heard if perchance they began to move in the coffin.

During the Enlightenment, some Jewish doctors encountered a troubling dilemma since their religious tradition required burial as soon as possible as a sign of respect. In 1612 Abraham Portoleone of Mantua in his will admonished his sons against burying him until 72 hours had elapsed. He wrote, "our sainted fathers were eager to hasten burial but do not marvel at what I ask for for not all scholars agree with one another."

In 1787 Dr. Markus Herz of Berlin published a pamphlet titled "On the premature burial of Jews" in which he agreed with a recently passed civil law that required waiting three days before internment lest an error be made. Dr. Herz asked, "Would it not be advisable to discontinue this practice and follow the example of our ethical and enlightened neighbors who watch over their dead for at least several days before burial?" Nevertheless, when Markus Herz died in 1803, he was buried promptly in a Jewish cemetery - with no bells attached.

In 1844 Edgar Allen Poe wrote a short story titled "The Premature Burial" in which the narrator, who suffers from severe cataplexy, has a morbid fear of being buried alive. After describing several recent instances of premature burials, he explained that "the stifling lack of air and fear of death combine with claustrophobia, darkness, and silence to form a terrifying ordeal that does not occur anywhere else on Earth." The narrator relates:

> *To be buried while still alive is, beyond question, the most terrific extreme which has ever fallen to the lot of mere mortality. That it has frequently, very frequently, so fallen will scarcely be denied by those who think. The boundaries which divide Life from Death are at best shadowy and vague. Who shall say where the one ends, and where the other begins?*

After "a distressing experience" in his own family, 19th century English social reformer William Tebb dedicated himself to stamping out the scourge of "death-counterfeits." By his estimate, in England and Wales alone some twenty-seven hundred people were annually "consigned to a living death…The thought of suffocation in a coffin is more terrible than that of torture on the rack, or burning at the stake … When we neglect precautions against a fate so terrible, our tears are little less than hypocrisy and our mourning is a mockery." And in 1896 William Tebb founded the London Association for the Prevention of Premature Burial.

All of this preceded the advent of modern diagnostic technology that, one would think, should have resolved the problem once and for all. But as we'll soon see has only muddied the waters. By the 1980s one could stop breathing, even have their heart stop beating, yet artificially be kept alive at least long enough until viable tissue could be transplanted from newly deceased donors. Because there weren't enough fresh hearts, lungs, kidneys and corneas that could be harvested, it became a practical matter to determine exactly when a potential candidate was legally dead.

THE HARVARD CRITERIA

Determination of death by strictly neurological criteria as an alternative to cardio-respiratory failure was first proposed in 1968 by a special committee at Harvard Medical School. They were concerned that obsolete criteria for defining death can lead to controversy in obtaining organs for transplantation and concluded that a diagnosis of brain death required irreversible, cessation of all functions of the *entire* brain. In 1981 the Harvard plan was adopted with some modifications into a model state law called the Uniform Determination of Death Act (UDDA.) It was approved by the National Conference of Commissioners on Uniform State Laws in cooperation with the American Medical Association, the American Bar Association and the President's Commission for the Study of Ethical Problems in Medicine and Biomedical and Behavioral Research and eventually was adopted by most states albeit with a few variations.

(Ad Hoc Committee to Examine the Definition of Brain Death. *JAMA,* (1968) 205: 85.

At about that same time, I was a fledgling physician in New Jersey and the UDDA seemed sensible to me - as it probably was to most physicians. However, I soon learned that things weren't so simple. I recall that I once had a female patient in her 40s who suffered a massive pulmonary embolism that caused such severe cerebral anoxia that she fulfilled the recently described neurologic criteria for "brain death." I gently asked her grief-stricken husband whether he'd be willing to donate her organs and although he was inclined to agree, first he'd have to consult his rabbi. They belonged to an Orthodox congregation in Paramus and, to my surprise, their rabbi's response was categorically no! Back then most Orthodox rabbis didn't recognize the brain death concept and their rabbi insisted that death can only be declared when breathing has stopped. Because this woman was being mechanically breathed she wasn't dead enough!

Although her husband was conflicted, eventually he agreed to permit organ donation in order to help others. Arrangements were made, the respirator was turned off, multiple organs were harvested and later the woman's family received many letters of thanks from grateful recipients. Rabbis were not the only ones troubled by these modern ideas. Some people argued that permanent loss of *higher* brain function - the ability to think - is what makes us "human" and without that capacity life isn't "worth" living. However, most others insisted on cessation of "whole-brain" function - not only the cerebral cortex but also the brain stem that controls vegetative functions including breathing. (In addition to Orthodox Jewish concerns, some Buddhists, Native Americans, and evangelical Protestants believe that someone is alive as long as their heart is beating.)

In 1985 I was appointed to New Jersey's newly formed Bioethics Commission, which functioned for about six years until government funding was eliminated, and brain death was among the issues that we discussed. I soon learned that everyone didn't understand things the way that I did. After a representative of an Orthodox Jewish organization (Agudath Yisrael) made a persuasive argument, we agreed that although the definition of death should be rooted in scientific knowledge, that life vs. death decisions also represent a societal choice that sometimes might be influenced by religion. The statute that was passed in 1991 by New Jersey's legislature contained a unique exemption: "Death cannot be declared in violation of an individual's religious beliefs." A physician should not declare someone dead if he or she, "has reason to believe… that it would violate the personal religious beliefs of the individual."

In effect, death became a legal *option* in New Jersey. In subsequent years religious exemptions to death by neurologic criteria occurred infrequently. A survey of New Jersey hospitals during the period between 2012 and 2016 turned up more than thirty cases of religious exemption, about half for Orthodox Jewish families. No requests for exemption were denied and during this same period there were 801 brain death donors in the state. The same year that New Jersey passed its brain death statute, New York State's highest court also adopted a religious exemption but this was through case law rather than statute and required only "reasonable accommodation" (24-72 hours) of personal beliefs.

(R.G. Son and S. Setta. Frequency of use of the religious exemption in New Jersey cases of determination of brain death. *BMC Medical Ethics* (2018) 19:76.)

The UDDA was intended to provide a comprehensive and medically sound basis for determining death in all situations, but in subsequent years the concept came under scrutiny and was the focus of legal challenges. Consider the case of Yechezkel Nakar who in 2017 while being treated at New York Presbyterian Hospital was diagnosed as being brain dead. When the hospital issued a death certificate over the objections of his orthodox Jewish family, Nakar was transferred to a different hospital where he received continued medical support for another 21 days until he met traditional diagnostic criteria. His wife filed a lawsuit in Brooklyn Supreme Court seeking to rescind the death certificate, presumably in order to make him eligible for insurance coverage for the intervening three weeks between brain death and cardiopulmonary death. In January 2019 the court ruled in favor of Nakar's family. (Incidentally, New Jersey's brain death law provides for continuation of health insurance coverage when there is a religious exemption.)

California and Illinois also require hospitals only to make "reasonable accommodations" to families' objections but it's not a blanket exemption as in New Jersey. In practice, most hospitals usually continue physiological support for a further 24 hours after declaring brain death. In New York this allows time for families to transfer the patient to New Jersey should they wish to do so. Indeed, "living corpses" have been flown in from much further - and not only Orthodox Jewish corpses.

LIFE AFTER DEATH

In 2013 Jahi McMath a thirteen year old Christian girl living in Oakland California suffered brain damage during throat surgery for sleep apnea but her parents refused to accept a diagnosis of brain death. In retrospect, they may have been correct and she might have been in a persistent vegetative state. After many months of medical-legal impasse, her body was flown to New Jersey where death is an "option." In total Jahi McMath's body survived for almost five years, during most of the time being cared for at home, and it continued to grow and develop with the onset of menarche. When her parents celebrated Jahi's 15th birthday they said "Our little sleeping beauty is doing good." They claimed that occasionally she moved a limb on command; more likely it was only a reflex. But in June 2018 Jahi developed internal bleeding due to kidney and liver failure and doctors, with her parent's consent, removed her from life support, allowing her to die by anyone's standards.

There've been several other cases of prolonged biologic life after neurological death. In 1998 pediatrician Alan Shewmon at UCLA claimed that he'd found 175 cases of somatic survival of a brain dead body that lasted at least a week; 28 cases for longer than a month, 17 cases longer than two months and 4 cases more than a year. Between 2005 and 2013, the ethics consultation service at the Cleveland Clinic reported thirteen requests for continued physiological support for a brain-dead patient. (Of these cases, three families cited their Orthodox Jewish faith, one referenced belief in God and another named their Islamic faith, reasons for the others were not stated.)

(Alan Shewmon. False-Positive Diagnosis of Brain Death Following the Pediatric Guidelines: Case Report and Discussion. *Journal of Child Neurology* (2017) 32: 1104.)

A JEWISH PERSPECTIVE

The traditional codifiers of Jewish law ruled that the primary test in determining whether a person is alive or dead involved the nose. This is based on a Biblical verse, "All in whose nostrils was the breath of the spirit of life" (Genesis 7:22), which implies that the "breath of the spirit of life" is what defines life. Although the Talmud doesn't directly discuss the matter, the question of determining death was addressed indirectly in a parable about what to do when a building collapses on Shabbat and it's uncertain if anyone alive is trapped underneath. Because of the principle of *pikuach nefesh*, in which saving a life takes priority over all else, the Talmud permits violating Shabbat in order to determine if anyone is alive under the rubble. It then asks which area of the victim's body one must examine to determine if he or she is alive or dead? The favored option was to uncover the buried victim from above until reaching the nose, seemingly indicating that the rescuer must look for signs of breathing.

One of my sons is a rabbi who for many years has served on the Law and Standards Committee of the Conservative movement that review difficult theological issues and establish guidelines. It seemed to him that the apnea test was a perfect compromise between Jewish tradition and the current state of medical expertise and in 2004 the law committee approved the proposal that permanent cessation of respiration established by the so-called "apnea test" met the standard of Jewish law - even superseding feathers and mirrors.

In this test the comatose patient is removed from the ventilator for about ten minutes and as the concentration of carbon dioxide in the blood rises It is a potent stimulus to respiration. If despite significant

CO2 elevation there's no measurable effort to breathe, than apnea is considered irreversible. Naturally, every medical test has a trade-off between sensitivity and specificity but death is unique in that it demands 100% specificity and 0% chance of a false-positive error. The apnea test is no exception and, it's been suggested that the test itself actually can be damaging to the brain. Moreover, some people may fail the apnea test and yet retain some brain stem functions. It's been reported that certain upper spinal cord injuries may prevent natural breathing yet the victim can remain conscious and very much alive. In other words, the body is capable of sustaining certain biologic activities even absent a functional brain stem.

(A. Joffe, et al. The Apnea Test: Rationale, Confounders and Criticism. *J. Child Neur.* (2010) 25: 1435.)

By now, the whole brain death standard is widely accepted but the issue continues to generate controversy. Some critics argue that more clarification is needed and, unless state laws are revised, that occasional lawsuits are likely to occur. A continuing challenge will be to educate the public about the differences between various kinds of brain damage and to make diagnostic tests as safe and reliable as possible. So far, brain death hasn't risen as an issue in the clinical context of COVID-19. Time will tell.

16

BRAIN STORM

COVID-19 has been a constant source of surprises and one of its least understood complications is what's generally referred to as a "cytokine storm." It's a malfunction of the body's own immune system that develops about a week after the onset of infection. In effect, the defense system turns on itself and goes into overdrive. In a subset of people it's this overcompensation that can lead to shock, respiratory failure and even death. Fortunately I averted that immunologic tempest but instead experienced a delayed intellectual disturbance - a *cognitive* storm if you will.

When they have nothing else to do, artists paint, musicians play and at least some historians write. I don't seriously propose that the corona virus itself caused my mental malaise, more likely it was a coping response to prolonged isolation and boredom. But whatever the initiating factor may have been, during my three month recuperation I experienced such a burst of pent-up creative energy that soon I'd collected enough historical digressions to fill this small book. Whereas cytokine storms may lead to the ICU, sometimes brain storms lead to the publisher.